The Elephant in the Room

Jonathan Waxman

The Elephant
in the Room

Stories About Cancer Patients
and their Doctors

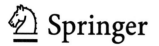 Springer

Author
Jonathan Waxman
Flow Foundation Professor
of Oncology
Imperial College London

ISBN 978-0-85729-894-2   e-ISBN 978-0-85729-895-9
DOI 10.1007/978-0-85729-895-9
Springer London Dordrecht Heidelberg New York

British Library Cataloguing in Publication Data
A catalogue record for this book is available from the British Library

Library of Congress Control Number: 2011938120

Printed on acid-free paper

Springer is part of Springer Science+Business Media (www.springer.com)

To Naomi, Thea and Freddie.

About the Author

Jonathan Waxman is Flow Foundation Professor of Oncology at Imperial College London. He founded The Prostate Cancer Charity, the first United Kingdom national organisation promoting research and patient support for this condition. He is a clinician who has helped develop new treatments for cancer, which are now part of standard practice. He is the author of eleven books on cancer, a book on medical negligence law and a novel, *The Fifth Gospel*. He directs a laboratory research group, and a clinical trial group. He has raised funds for the building of the Hammersmith Cancer Centre whose spirit aims to combine the best of conventional and alternative therapies. He helped establish an All Party Parliamentary Group to improve cancer treatment and rationalise cancer research throughout the UK. He has developed and led successful and unsuccessful media campaigns to rationalise cancer treatments and change government health policy.

Beginnings: Jimmy's Gift

This book started life as a conversation between the writer, J G Ballard, and his doctor. I was his doctor. The conversations were to be about life and death.

Jimmy had prostate cancer, and the plan for the book had reached a point where an outline had been sketched and the content planned. I had put to Jimmy the concept of a project about cancer. I had suggested the idea of a jointly written book based around the relationship between a patient and his specialist. Jimmy and I were hugely excited about the idea of the book. We intended to spend time together talking about the impact of cancer on his life, what it really meant to be a patient, the interactions between doctors and patients, what the doctor and the patient really thought about, and what the doctor really meant when he spoke to patients. This exchange was to be bound by a thread that took in our journeys through life. It was to be a contemporaneous account of two lives intertwined and interlinked.

So, that's what had been planned, and the plan was bound to extend beyond its loosely set outlines and borders.

Jimmy set about writing a book proposal.

But before our project could be realized, darkness struck, and Jimmy became too poorly to think about writing. And so the book was never written, and the proposal languished in my filing cabinets until the moment of Jimmy's memorial service. This celebration of Jimmy's life was held on the top floor of the Tate, with great views over the Thames, exotic canapés, and a gathering of friends and family who had come to celebrate Jimmy's life. We sat together, listening to speeches that brought together all the parts of Jimmy's world, speeches from Jimmy's wonderful daughters, writers, friends, film producers, and the marvellously self-effacing, baseball hat-wearing, Stephen Spielberg.

As Jimmy's treating doctor I had been invited to close with a tribute to Jimmy. At the end of my talk, as I stood in sunlight at the lectern, I was left with the feeling that somehow I'd let Jimmy down by not completing our project.

I'd had a history with Jimmy that antedated his illness. We had met many years before he was ill, when I had looked after one of his dear friends who had breast cancer. That was in the 1990s, and I had just completed work on my third and as yet unpublished novel, to write was my big dream.

I decided to impose upon Jimmy and exploit the contact that had been made with him. I asked him to read my book. I put the book in the post, and sent it to him on a Friday for comments, with apologies for imposing on him. He read my book over the weekend, and I received a blue biro letter from him on Tuesday morning, expressing interest, and suggesting that he might send the book to his agent Margaret Hanbury if I would allow him to do so. Well, of course I would allow him to do so, and the introduction led to the publication of my first novel, an event ranking a great deal below the arrival of children in consequence, but still of some enormous excitement to me.

Events in my own life took a poor turn, and creativity took second place to child care and earning a living. In the place where I earned a living I met Jimmy again. He had become ill and I was so pleased to be able to help him as he had helped me. He was transformed by treatment and from being dreadfully sick, and in considerable pain, he became remarkably well.

And Jimmy produced 'Miracles of Life'.

When in remission of his cancer, Jimmy would come to clinic every month and, on many occasions he would ask me about my writing. He would embarrass me by telling me that I really should get writing again. He'd say …

"You really should you know."

And his right hand would give emphasis to his comment with a curving karate chop that cut the cold consulting room air and entirely seized up the conversation.

And my embarrassment would increase further.

These exchanges caused me great discomfort. Some of the discomfort was due to the fact that I was not being creative, and possibly could be, and the rest of the discomfort was due to the fact that I couldn't break the barrier of patient/doctor relationship to explain to him the reasons why I could not be creative. I wished somehow that I could break the barrier, and explain to him why it was that I had failed to come up to standard and produced another little effort.

I looked again at our outline after his memorial service, and felt that somehow and in some way this was his gift to me, the stimulus for a book on cancer. With his loss our collaboration could never be realised, what had been conversation was now a monologue. In its creation the book comes from my life as a cancer doctor, its errors and idiocies are mine, and my intentions and ambitions are to explain and guide.

I have written about the patient and his cancer and described what the doctor feels, described what the doctor really thinks as he talks to his patient. The faults and fractures in these stories are mine, but I have done my best for the love of a great man.

Acknowledgements

The writer of this book acknowledges his debt to his patients and to his teachers, Dr E Emery, Dr John Hickman, Professor Ernie Huehns, Dr Barry Hulme, Dr P Kidner, Professors T A Lister, R T Oliver and J S Malpas, to his friend Ian Fiertag who was the first to explain to him how patients might feel, to his agent Margaret Hanbury, his publisher Denise Roland, to Jimmy Ballard, Claire Walsh, Brian Clarke, Harry Woolf, Raoul Coombes, Adrian Dannatt, and Sandie Coward, and to the editorial skills and encouragement of Naomi Heaton.

Introduction

Cancer is the elephant in the room, a grim, grey ghost, draped in rags, dripping slime, hunched behind the sofa waiting on his time. And the elephant is readying himself for that moment when he will leap out to meet you in your unsuspecting moments, an ice axe, chain saw moment that you knew would be yours at some time.

But somehow even though rationally you knew that there would be a time, you never thought that time would come. You thought and you hoped that it would be your fate somehow, if God was good, and there was a God, that you would die in your own safe bed in the middle of a dark night in the depths of your deepest sleep, die in greatest old age, in the calm comfort and bright love of your family.

What evidence is there that God is good, when that nice doctor chap with the gentle face and soft manners has told you, that unfortunately,

"The tests have shown …"

What evidence is there that there is any God at all, when God in his omnipotence has created a fate that for you is …

"… a cancer."

So you go through all the tests, the biopsies and the scans, the little blows and the large discomforts, the surgery and the chemotherapy, the radiotherapy and the sickness, the pain and the sadness, over weeks or months, and at the end of it there is a stiletto silence as you wait for the words that tell you that you will live or you will die.

For one in three of us in the industrialised world, this is our fate but the odds are not on death, they are on life. In the United Kingdom 150,000 people survive cancer each year.

But how can a patient be optimistic about his prospects for survival when he thinks he's tramping through the killing fields?

Optimism is grounded in the evolution of cancer treatment which rides the red hot rocket of modern science. Advances in treatment have developed from the incredible progress that has been made in our understanding of the molecular biology of cancer, an understanding that has thankfully been exploited by pharmaceutical companies.

Pharmaceutical companies are driven by the hunger of the stock market and fuelled by the need for profit. The great corporations, the GSKs and the Astrazenecas, the Mercks and the Eli Lillys, the Sanofiaventises and the Pfizers have given us drugs, great drugs. May their shareholders be blessed forever! Greed has been very good for cancer. Where 50 years ago we had no treatments for cancer we now have many drugs. The pharmaceutical companies have brought us gifts, chemotherapy and targeted therapies, antibodies and computer modelled molecular treatments.

Cancer and its treatment has become highly specialised with a language and a life that is complex and technological. The translation of its processes, the explanation of its ways is beyond comprehension, and many patients revert to the primitive and seemingly irrational to cope. When they do so, they are exploited by the black-hearted and the craven, the unprincipled and the merely fanatic. The irrational takes hold of the materially successful, the politicians and movie moguls, the professors and chief executives. The irrational takes hold of the materially less successful, the unemployed and the labourer, the postman and the milkman. The masters of our universe and the people in the queues at the job centres are conjoined twins in their ignorance; all are lost stumbling through the mists of a Cancer Haze led by a squint eyed soothsayer with a megaphone preaching an occult sermon.

For all, from the most learned to the ignorant, from the rational to the irrational, lives are changed forever by their schemes for dealing with their disease. The ways that they manage their cancers are not the ways in which they have ruled their lives but come from a complete lack of understanding of their conditions. Their methods are brave attempts to seize back control of lives cast adrift, adrift in the cold oceans, locked in by sea monsters and serpents. Intelligent men and women lay on putrid poultices and shove lamb serum enemas up their bottoms. Why do they do these things? Why is it that in a land where all hope is lost witchcraft takes a hold?

When we have been told what is wrong with us so many of us cannot understand what it is that we have heard and we go to the Internet and search the bookshelves to find a way through, a way that tells us what it is that we are going through. But there is no simple guide that takes us through the Cancer Badlands. What I hope to do in this book is empower the cancer patient through plain language and the examples of others to find their path through cancer diagnosis and treatment. I have written about cancer through the lives of patients, showing the way by explaining how doctors as well as patients think.

So this book would be the spark that gives people who feel no hope a chance to see that the place they are in is the start of their journey, and not its end. From my life as a cancer doctor, come stories, true stories.

Contents

Chapter 1
Rick's Big Adventure

"We've got this young guy here … Can you sort him out?"

This is doctor talk and doctor talk can be translated into a form of English that is comprehensible to normal folk … And the translation is …

'We are completely at a loss and we haven't a clue what to do.'

"He presented with back pain to his GP and the X-rays showed erosion at T12."

This can be translated too and the translation is …

'He has a cancer that has spread to his spine and is eating away at his twelfth thoracic vertebra, one of the bones that form the spinal column.'

"So we got a scan and it showed a large mass arising out of the kidney, extending to and eroding the spine. The biopsy showed a renal cell cancer. He's a really nice guy, and his wife is a nurse."

There is an element of a sales pitch when patients are referred from one doctor to another. The sales pitch gives the doctor status. If the patient is exceptional then that doctor will be exceptional because he has been chosen to look after an exceptional patient.

And as it happens the patient is exceptional, a decent, generous, sensitive and altruistic man!

Rick had gone to his GP with backache and his doctor had sensed that unlike most people who complain of backache this was a symptom that required more than paracetamol and

J. Waxman, *The Elephant in the Room*,
DOI 10.1007/978-0-85729-895-9_1,
© Springer-Verlag London Limited 2012

reassurance … it needed investigation; it needed a proper sort out.

Rick was relatively short and slight, he invariably dressed in jeans and a T-shirt, and usually wore his hair in a pony tail. Rick was thoughtful and sensitive, and carried his gentleness before him on a banner of smiles. He was constitutionally incapable of travelling more than ten yards from his front door without a copy of *the Guardian*.

The GP had looked at Rick and had seen and sensed that there was something seriously wrong. Rick looked too pale, his pallor too much even for the most radical of socialists living through a hard South West London winter in a Conservative constituency. Rick looked too drawn, too sucked in at the cheeks. To his doctor, Rick's appearance could not be ascribed merely to the stresses of life as an inner city schoolteacher. To his doctor, Rick had the look of being bothered by something, something that had more than the usual volume and amplitude of the ordinary backache.

There are a series of investigations that can be done to sort out the reasons for the sort of pain that Rick had mentioned to his doctor. They start with simple tests, and as the results of these tests become available, further more complex investigations are booked. The simple tests are basic blood tests that give an idea of how the liver and kidneys are working, and tell the doctor whether the patient is anaemic. These blood test results are assessed with two additional tests that show if the patient is well or unwell. These additional tests seem like medieval magic. They are called 'ESR' and 'CRP'. ESR is the rate at which red blood cells sink. In the lab a tube of the patient's blood is set up and the rate at which the red cells settle in the tube over the course of an hour is measured. If the red cells sink quickly, to reveal a big expanse of clear yellowish plasma, settled on a short column of red cells, then the patient is sick. If the red cells fall slowly then the patient is well! It is magic but the explanation is as with most magic, simple, illuminating and reveals further magical mysteries. CRP is an inflammatory marker… it's a protein that increases when the body is stressed by the presence of cancer or infection.

Rick watched as the nurse in the GP's clinic sunk what seemed like an enormous needle into the veins of his forearm. He desisted from saying to the nurse that she was taking a whole armful, which was just as well because she had heard the line over 10,000 times and had sworn to her husband earlier in the day, that if she heard the phrase again she'd kick the next patient who said '… a whole armful …' or eat the chair that he was sitting on.

Rick's blood test results showed him to be anaemic and to have a raised ESR, which prompted the doctor to feel that he had been right in taking Rick's symptoms seriously. The doctor had also given Rick an X-ray request form for films of the spine, and Rick made his way to the local hospital for the X-ray. In the X-ray department, Rick was shown into a changing cubicle and given a gown to wear, one of those open flappy things that gape at the back, an item of clothing that must have been maliciously designed by a horny bug eyed red nosed devil to provide patients' private parts with intimate access to the cold, cold wind that scuffs along the corridors of Tundra Hospital, SE21.

Rick lay on the X-ray couch, and as if a dispassionate observer of self, noted that lying down made his pain worse. X-rays were taken and the images viewed on a screen by radiologist. When something very abnormal is seen on an X-ray, then the doctors who specialise in interpreting X-rays, who are called radiologists, fax or phone their reports to the GP or consultant who have requested the X-rays; it's part of their duty of care to do so. Rick's films were particularly horrible and the radiologist's report was faxed the same day to the GP.

The X-ray of Rick's back showed that part of his spine had a hole in it. The twelfth thoracic spine wasn't a nice white bracelet of bone, it wasn't solid and substantial; it was ragged and fragile. Instead of normal bone the X-ray showed that there was a large nip taken from the edge of the vertebra. It was as if a mongoose with metal teeth had nibbled lumps from the edges of his spine, and termites in a hurry had burrowed through its central mass.

Rick had been given a repeat, routine follow up appointment at his GP's practice but when the fax came tumbling through, his doctor knew that he had to be seen as soon as possible and referred urgently for a specialist opinion. His doctor felt dread in his heart for Rick. He knew what the result meant, knew the suffering that he would go through, understood its significance for Rick and Rachel. He rang Rick on his mobile.

"It's your GP Rick, it's Jim Barber ..."

"I'm in a class right now doctor, please could you hold on for a moment ... please ..."

Rick stepped outside of his classroom, kids staring, heart pounding, everything pounding.

"Go ahead doctor."

"Rick. Can you come up and see me in the surgery tonight please?"

"It's bad news doc, isn't it?"

" ...'fraid so Rick ..." there was nothing else that could be said.

In the surgery that evening Rick and Rachel held hands as the doctor explained that unfortunately it was likely that Rick had a tumour pressing on his spine.

'Yes,' thought Rick ...

'Unfortunately.'

Rick toyed with the word in his mind, it came and went and then rolled back again, growing in size. It was all that his brain seemed to be able to do; all that could be done was to roll the word backwards and forwards and then sometimes sideways so that all thought, all thinking was centred on ...

'Unfortunately'.

Yes.

'Unfortunately'.

There was only that echoing word and no emotion.

'UNFORTUNATELY.'

There was only the word, and then Rick thought wryly, that in the end as in the beginning there is only the word ... apparently. And he smiled. And smiled again realising that he was off on a tangent and really should concentrate and what was it that he should be concentrating on? Oh yes the word 'Unfortunately', and he was brought back into the surgery by sobbing and a certain spasmodic, jerking, tugging on his hand.

He noticed that his doctor looked very uncomfortable and heard Rachel crying. It all seemed at a distance; everything that was going on was a space away from him.

"We'll refer you to hospital Rick."

The referral took him to his local hospital where a consultation, blood tests and CT scans followed. Nobody gave him anything for the pain, but then again Rick hadn't asked for anything so how should the doctors know what was wanted or needed? But actually, Rick didn't want any painkillers. He felt that they would only mask what was going on inside him and he wanted to know what it was that was happening to him.

After the scans had been carried out … rather quickly … Rick had thought and thought with some satisfaction, knowing that the NHS was actually, yes actually, functioning very well indeed … he was told that he would,

" … need a biopsy to find out what it was that was wrong with him."

The consultant explained, crossing and uncrossing his legs as if in emphasis of the details of the procedure.

So it was another trip to the X-ray Department.

A radiologist in surgical scrubs leaned over his belly … Rick's belly that is, not the radiologist's belly, Rick's belly, skin shrouded in surgical drapes, a small square of framed, pale flesh exposed. The radiologist flourished a vicious looking needle, inspected it myopically, pulled the plunger in and out, and whistled 'Land of Hope and Glory', the glory Rick noted, being rather flat.

'Could be worse' Rick mused,

'Might be 'Vicious', and we wouldn't want that would we?'

The consultant leaned his elbow on Rick's belly and Rick tried not to wince.

"I am going to inject local anaesthetic so you will only feel me pushing, you won't feel any pain."

Rick was unconvinced.

"This is a Truecut needle."

The needle was rather too flamboyantly exhibited and Rick felt sure that the radiologist's flourishes were a trifle excessive given the job in hand.

" … and I am going to use it to take a small specimen from your tummy. We'll look at it under the microscope and hopefully find out what's wrong."

The radiologist leaned more heavily on Rick's belly, and peered at a computer screen.

"I can see what I am doing and where I am going inside your belly, by using this piece of kit and looking at the images on my screen."

The radiologist showed Rick a piece of apparatus that looked like a microphone.

" … it's like the system that's used to look at babies in the womb."

"You mean ultrasound doctor," said Rick.

"Exactly."

Said the doctor, and smeared cold jelly onto Rick's belly, without any explanation as to what he was doing.

'Odd that!' thought Rick.

'In any other situation I might either be very worried about what was going to happen next or hoping that I might be getting a rather wonderful massage!'

The doctor leaned over Rick's belly and concentrated on his probe and then looked up at his screen. Rick noticed that his belly button involuntarily twitched away from the jelly and probe, a belly button that clearly wished to have nothing to do with the process and wanted to be back home cosy and warm, sitting with its owner, Rick, tucked up with a nice gin toddy in the belly's flat in Kingston.

'It's all right for you mate.' thought Rick,

'You're just a belly button, and you have not a single thought in your head because you haven't got a head just in case you had forgotten that you hadn't got a head. What about me? I have got a head. I think. You, you miserable button of flesh, you haven't a single thought in your ridiculous existence, so shut up and stop fidgeting.'

The radiologist viewing his computer screen saw that the mass of tumour in Rick's belly was intimately connected to major blood vessels, draped around Rick's aorta and vena cava. He knew that if his needle took a trip and hit the vessels, he would encounter a gallon of blood and a large compensation claim from Rick's widow. He held steady and advanced his needle slowly, slowly, catchee catchee …

His friend the needle pushed in through the skin of Rick's belly and a shower of white waves appeared on the screen, flickered and then coalesced into an image of dolphins flicking through a dark sea. Well that's what it seemed like to Rick when actually to the more professionally soignée, it was an image of his tumour mass curled perilously around Rick's aorta.

"That's it! I've got it."

The radiologist smiled and yanked out the needle. He peered at it and then discarded the needle's contents into a small plastic pot. Rick saw blood swirl from the needle around the container. The radiologist checked on his screen to make sure that there was no internal fountain of bright blood denoting catastrophic haemorrhage, angulating his probe so that he could sweep though Rick's belly, and check for disasters. All though was calm.

A bubble of bright blood blebbed up from the insertion point of the needle in Rick's belly and the nurse assisting the radiologist leaned over and dabbed a cotton wool swab on Rick's skin and pressed. The radiologist elbow was removed from Rick's soft parts much to Rick's relief. And Rick thought

'That elbow had been by far the worst thing of the whole procedure …

'That biopsy was not so bad really. But that elbow …! Hope that I won't have to go through that elbow thing again!'

Rick chuckled and the clinical team stared at him, doctor, radiographer, and nurse gawping at the lunatic laughing.

Ten days went by, ten anxious days, during which the specimen taken from Rick's tumour was processed. The sample was fixed in formalin, cut in wafer thin sections, stuck on a microscope slide, stained, and then peered at by a pathologist who identified the type of tumour that Rick was suffering from.

And at the end of the ten days Rick and Rachel sat once more with the consultant to whom they had been referred by their GP. Then with leg crossing and the occasional splutter, the doctor explained that,

" ... Actually, yes actually, I am actually very sorry to have to tell you that there is bit of trouble I am afraid ... and that I will need to refer you to a colleague who will I am sure sort things out."

But as he spoke the consultant thought,

'I can't believe I've said that, the poor chap is absolutely stuffed.'

There was not much more than this in terms of an explanation and Rick wasn't minded to go through things all at once. He didn't want to know everything at once, just a fact at a time would do him nicely.

The consultant continued,

'Any questions?'

... But really, really ... really hoping that there were no questions because it was getting towards the end of the clinic, and he hadn't had any coffee. And ... and, he had got a rather bad hangover. God, he had a bad hangover, and he was worried that his wife knew that he was having an affair with the senior sister on his ward, who was the beautiful cause of today's hangover. God, she was beautiful. And she, she, she ... and she could cook ...

The consultant seemed to have become silent for a moment and Rachel interrupted the silence.

"So, then, an appointment will be sent to us or should we phone up and make an appointment?"

The consultant seemed startled by the question, which worried Rachel.

'Oh Lord!' thought the consultant,

'Christ. What was it that I was saying to these poor people?'

"Oh yes ... I will refer you and an appointment should get to you but just in case it doesn't, do ring my colleague, who will be looking after you, he's called ... Professor Dickinson, and you couldn't be in better hands."

So Rick and Rachel went home. They waited until the door of the flat was shut and they'd had a stiff one before discussing what a diagnosis of 'A bit of trouble' actually meant. They knew though that the consultant had implied that things were serious and being not the daftest people in the world realised that serous meant life threatening and adding up the sum total of a lump in the belly and 'A bit of trouble', came to view that Rick had cancer. They poured themselves another drink.

But why was it that the doctor hadn't given a proper diagnosis?

Well ... who does like giving bad news? We all like good news; we hate the repercussions of bad tidings. Who wants to think about death and destruction? Who is it that wishes to confront the patient with a limited survival chance? Who wants to witness tears and heartbreak? So you could just about understand how it was that the consultant didn't want to be frank with Rick and Rachel. You could understand his lack of clarity, but understanding an action doesn't mean that the action can be condoned.

Meanwhile the days went by and Rick and Rachel received an appointment through the post to see Professor Dickinson who apparently was ...

... a consultant in Oncology.

The appointment had come remarkably quickly, so quickly that it made them wonder if Rick's case was very serious. The case was serious but the appointment's speed was the result of government health care priorities, and not to do with the urgency of Rick's case. The government has set guidelines as to target dates for appointments, scans and treatment. Failure to fulfil targets results in a financial penalty being applied to the failing hospital.

'Oncology Outpatients!' mused Rick,

'So it is serious then. Oncology, that means Cancer.'

Rachel turned her head away from him; she didn't want him to see that she was crying.

Meanwhile Rick's case had been reviewed at an MDT meeting. This three letter acronym stands for 'Multidisciplinary Team'. There are a lot of TLA's in the NHS. Rick's story had been presented to a panel of senior and junior doctors who represented the different specialty services involved in the management of cancer patients. The specialisations included pathology and radiology, surgery and oncology. The meeting was held in the presence of nurses, clerical staff, and students. The panel had looked at the microscopic appearance of the samples taken from Rick's lump, and reviewed his scans. The future management of his condition was discussed, debated and planned. A decision was made about the course of his treatment and a note made of how that treatment was to proceed. That note was kept as a record within Rick's clinical records together with a note of the time course of the decision making process, which included appointment times and length of time for scans and for treatment to be completed.

The panel had seen that Rick had an enormous lump the size and shape of a deformed butternut squash, curling out from his right kidney, the origin of his cancer and reaching into and around the back of his abdomen with roots and tendrils that grasped at Rick's spine. They considered that there might be a danger to Rick of that tumour expanding to eat further into his spine and spread through the bone into the central cavity that contained the spinal cord that the spinal column protected. This would lead to paralysis if left untreated. The MDT had collectively come to the view that Rick needed radiotherapy treatment to prevent the paralysis.

So a radiotherapist sent an appointment for Rick to be seen in his clinic. Rick and Rachel sat with him whilst he explained the reasons for treatment and how the treatment worked.

Rick embarked on a course of radiotherapy treatment to reduce the risk of the cancer causing paralysis. It was a treatment that was given daily for two weeks. The radiotherapy made him feel a little tired and the fatigue became worse as the treatment progressed. The doctors reviewing him told him to…

'Take a snooze in the afternoons. The tiredness will pass. There's absolutely no point fighting it.'

Rick liked the public school accent. For some reason it was a comfort.

'Maybe it's the authority figure I'm responding to?' he thought.

Rick wondered about that.

'Can't square that with reading *The Guardian*.' And he giggled silently.

Rick felt a little sick as well as exhausted.

"It's radiation sickness ... that will pass too. You might get a little diarrhoea as well. Have some pills, they'll help you."

They did but they made him constipated, so much so, that Rick wasn't sure what was worse ... the constipation or the nausea. He decided to take a rain check on all medicines and gave up every tablet, the blue ones and the white ones, the green and the pink and hoped that with time all things would pass, along with the diarrhoea, and he giggled again as he thought about the passing of diarrhoea.

Radiotherapy treatment had finished and now it was time for Rick to be reviewed. He sat in clinic with Rachel and listened to the registrar talk.

"We've considered your case."

'That's a start.' thought Rick.

"And we want to send you to see another doctor who works in our department."

Rick nodded. And panicked ...

'They've given up on me. Why is everyone passing me on?'

This sort of sentiment is common. Patients get used to one doctor and take confidence in that constancy. The referral of a patient to another doctor might imply that the referring doctors have given up, that the case is difficult and that there is no hope. But that's not quite the right sort of logic. It is a good sign, a sign of openness and confidence in your own practice if you are prepared to enlist the help of other teams of clinicians. Patients aren't property, though they are often regarded as such, and the best patient care is usually shared patient care.

"You see there have been great changes in the way that cancer of the kidney ..."

Rick felt himself twitch. That was the first time that anyone had ever mentioned the word 'cancer' to him. Even though he knew that he had cancer, it still came as quite a shock to hear the word enunciated.

'It's funny,' he thought,

'How you can know you have cancer, yet when the cancer word is mentioned for the first time, it's like the shock of knowing begins again.'

"So if you could come back to the Department on Wednesday morning, the professor will see you and explain everything."

But Rick had already been issued with an appointment to see the professor, an appointment that had been delayed by radiotherapy treatment.

However regardless of any mix up as to who would be seeing whom and when, Rick looked forward to the explanation that the professor would give him. Which duly came from the thin lips of a shortish chap with curly hair who smiled a lot, smiled rather inappropriately at the wrong parts of the conversation where possibly a more serious attitude should have prevailed.

"You know it's a wonderful time to have kidney cancer!"

Rick found this remarkable.

The professor went on to explain.

"You see we have new treatments for the condition that come from our understanding of the molecular biology of kidney cancer."

The professor had noticed that Rick and Rachel were sensitive and intelligent people. He tried to explain the molecular biology thing in terms that people who had no understanding of science might understand. He understood that almost every word of medical language was incomprehensible to people who hadn't been medically trained and that a sort of slumping quietness came over intelligent men and women when he tried to explain how things worked in the world where he worked.

"Kidney cancers are the result of abnormal growth of what used to be normal tissue because of the activity of something called an oncogene."

The professor noticed that familiar glazed look sweep slowly across Rick and Rachel's collective brows.

'Uh-oh!' he thought.

'We'll have to go even more basic.'

"I take it you don't have the foggiest about what I am trying to explain!"

Rick and Rachel agreed that they were befogged.

"An oncogene is called an oncogene because it is the genetic signal that leads to a cancer growing in normal tissues. It can do so by stimulating the growth of a tumour directly or by allowing the tumour to grow because other genes are switched on. Uncontrolled growth is the characteristic of cancer."

It was little wonder that people had trouble understanding him. Trouble is that science is complex … and medical science is just not the sort of thing that you get to understand after a night in a pub with a medical student, unless that medical student is really good looking. Trouble is that even the most basic of words that are used by scientists to explain things are built on layers of complexity layered on even more layers of complexity.

"In patients with kidney cancer there is a mutation in a gene present on the third pair of chromosomes. This mutation may be inherited or more commonly it comes as a new mutation, which results from an unknown cause."

"So, professor, my genes have gone wrong?"

"One of your genes Rick."

"In kidney cancer this change, this mutation, leads to a decrease in a cell protein that changes the cell's perception of the amount of oxygen that it is receiving.

"As a result …"

The professor noted with some relief that Rick and Rachel were both following his explanation.

'What a relief …' he thought,

'Someone understands me. Wish it was like that at home! Aren't they nice. I like them.'

" … As a result the kidney cell makes more of a receptor on its surface, a receptor that tells the tissues in which it is embedded that it wants more oxygen. The tissues respond by manufacturing blood vessels to supply the cell with more oxygen carried by the blood stream. But the down side to this increased oxygenation is that the cell has now developed the characteristics of a cancer cell. It's made its own blood supply. It's growth has become out of control … it has become a cancer."

"And the upside?" asked Rachel.

"I have had enough of downsides for six life times!"

"Quite enough!" commented the professor and smiled again.

"The upside is that because we know the molecular reasons for the tumour's development we have been able to design treatments that are designed to focus on the abnormality that has caused the cancer. We have produced treatments that target these molecular changes and shrink the tumour."

"That's the first good news, the first upside we've heard for quite a while."

"And … they work … about 40 to 60% of patients improve."

" … and the downside?"

"Good question. How did you know there is a catch?"

"Stands to reason."

"The catch … it's that there are organisations called the Primary Care Trusts. We have to apply to your PCT in order to get approval for the use of the new drug."

"What's that?"

"Guess that you have heard of NICE?"

Rachel and Rick both nodded.

"As you probably both know NICE makes decisions about the cost effectiveness of a new drug and the Government follows that NICE decision on whether that new treatment should be prescribed by doctors and used by patients. NICE is famous for taking a huge length of time to make up its mind and we have a real problem about the way that it comes to its decisions. The trouble is that NICE uses a subjective rating scale that is completed by people who may not have cancer or indeed any illness, to come to a view about the cost benefit of a new treatment.

"Anyway I mustn't go on … but … in the meantime whilst NICE is deliberating, it's up to the local PCTs … the organisations that pay for the drugs to make up their minds as to whether or not they are prepared to fund the drugs that could make you better."

"What do you mean professor? Isn't it sufficient that an expert who has been trained for 30 years should say that we need the drugs?"

"The simple answer is 'No'. I have to fill in an application form to your PCT in order to allow me to use the drug. It's a complex form."

"How long does it take to get this sorted out?"

"I promise I will complete the form in the next day or so but it will take the PCT at least two weeks to come to a view."

"Who are the people that make the decisions in the PCT?" asked Rachel, edging forward in her seat and flushing.

"They are GPs, public health doctors and pharmacists."

"And what do they know about cancer?"

"Not a lot in my opinion."

"So these non-specialists are making decisions about issues that they know very little about?"

"You've got it on the button."

"That's outrageous."

"Yup and it's outrageous 150 times around the country. There are 150 PCTs and they are all making local decisions about whether or not a patient deserves a drug. The PCT's decision is based on whether or not the patient and his circumstances are exceptional enough for that patient to be allowed to have the new treatment, and whether that drug is worth it on the basis of its efficacy and cost…"

The professor warmed to his favourite subject … the horrors of local autonomy … how the devolution of decision making absolved government from responsibility for health … if they didn't watch out he'd go on about the cost of the PCTs, the £5 billion each year that it took to run the system. But then it wasn't going to help the patient was it, to go into detail?

"Look I'll do my best, you have my word. Let's make a provisional appointment for review in three weeks and hopefully we will be sorted out by then. If we hear earlier I'll call you."

At the end of his clinic the professor returned to his office, sat down at his desk, and opened up the application form.

"Buggery I hate these forms. Billions of blistering blue barnacles, how I hate these bloody forms."

The professor scratched, shuffled, searched eBay, looked at the BBC news web page, and then grumbling and swearing, swearing much more than he should, concentrated on completing the application form to the PCT requesting the drug that he and all the other doctors in his specialty would want to prescribe Rick.

Three weeks later the professor walked in to his secretary's office and said,

"Have you had any correspondence from the PCT about Rick's sunitinib?"

"Nope. What are you expecting? Miracles? Don't you know yet what they are like?"

"I think I do but ... there's always hope."

"There may be hope but not there Sunshine!"

So the professor emailed the hospital pharmacist whose responsibility it was to deal with the PCTs. He asked her to make the enquiry about when a decision might be expected from the PCT. She let him know that the decision had been made but they were waiting in the PCT for the letter about the decision to be typed. The professor asked if the letter could be faxed to the hospital because he knew how long letters took to navigate through the system.

Some three days later the decision letter was issued, faxed and read. The reading material did not make for happiness. The decision of the panel which is based upon patient exceptionality was that the drug could not be given.

Now what exactly is 'exceptionality'? The professor had had to make the case that Rick and his circumstances were exceptional. The definition of exceptionality is of course a subjective judgement. We are all exceptional. The basis for the professor's case for Rick's exceptionality was Rick's youth, his life expectancy if untreated, the fact that the new treatment had been demonstrated to have efficacy, and that all previously available treatments had little chance of working.

"Well stuff that and f … them. How can they do that? I am bloody well going to phone them. What are they on?"

"Can I speak to someone that makes the decision about …?"

"I am afraid they are in a meeting right now."

"May I leave my number …?"

"Yes, they will call you back."

They didn't, so the professor tried again, and got through to …

"You can appeal the panel's decision."

"Great … how do I do that?"

"You can re-apply."

"But if I do that I will only be giving you the same information as before, the stuff that I have already given you."

"How long does the appeal process take?"

"Should be a couple of weeks."

"But that makes it more than 6 weeks … what about the patient?"

"OK then we can set up a Virtual Appeals Panel."

" … And how long will that take?"

"Couple of days."

Three days had gone by and the professor had not heard the panel's decision. Time to call again, to find that the panel hadn't actually 'virtualised'

… So another call and after hearing the familiar …

"She's in a meeting"

… several times, the professor finally got through to find that the meeting still hadn't taken place. By this time the professor had found out that the virtual panel consisted of two GPs, neither of whom of course had specialist training in the area of cancer medicine. He was not at a loss to understand how non-specialists could be empowered to make such decisions, as he had grey hair and had dealt with the system for aeons.

And finally he found the panel chair and learnt from her that the decision had been positive.

His secretary called Rick and Rachel and let them know that they had won. The professor liked to give his secretary the good news jobs. It made her day better. The bad news jobs ... they tended to be face to face, no secretary.

So the next day came and the professor sat in the clinic with Rick and Rachel once more.

"So, we can start then ...?"

"Yes. Now I'd like to tell you about the side effects of treatment."

The professor looked up to observe the expressions on their faces as he began to speak about the list of side effects likely to be caused by the treatment. Now, doctors do not have to list all the side effects that a treatment may cause, just the common ones. The reason why they don't have to list all side effects is pretty obvious ... the list can last hours! If the patient wants to know what problems the drugs prescribed can cause he can read the information on the product data list that he receives when he picks up his treatment from pharmacy. Open the box and it's all there ... in the box.

The professor was watching their expressions to ensure that the messages that he was going to give them about the side effects of treatment were understood. He was waiting for that fluorescent glimmer, the spark of the 'on switch' on the light bulb over their toupees, the flash of insight shimmering above his patient's head. And failing that he would write down what it was that the patient had to watch out for because it was really important that they understood what he was saying. Because Rick could die if they didn't understand.

Now the treatment that the professor had taken so much trouble to get for his patient is designed to stop the growth of the blood vessels induced by the cancer. But blood vessels grow everywhere in the body, and the same cellular signals that provide new blood vessels for the cancer are also present in normal cells and lead to new blood vessel formation in skin and gut and just about everywhere else. So naturally, because this process is not specific to the cancer, and because the treatment given doesn't just stop blood vessels forming around the cancer but stops blood vessels growing everywhere, there can be side effects that are caused by the treatment that are really significant. These tend to be most devastating where tissues are thin and very actively dividing and so in need of new blood vessels to support their structure.

So, this growth of blood vessels can be inhibited in other body organs … in organs sited almost anywhere. But the important place where this inhibition can happen in terms of the danger from treatment is in the gut. If the guts' blood vessel formation is significantly halted then the wall of the gut can become short of blood and die. If gut dies then a hole can form. This can result in peritonitis, where the gut's contents, the acids and partially digested food, the faeces and bile, spills out into the abdomen. Or there can be catastrophic bleeding from the gut. Both of these conditions, if they are not recognised at an early point can progress and lead to the patient's death and this is not what the doctors want!

This was definitely not what the professor wanted, having seen catastrophe happen and a dearly beloved patient die as a result of an unrecognised bleed. There's nothing like seeing an exsanguinating patient in Casualty surrounded by her weeping family, nothing like seeing your patient die from a side effect of the treatment that you have prescribed, to chasten the heart.

The professor's chastening experience had occurred at a time when doctors had not been clued in to the toxicity of sunitinib. The use of new drugs requires experience and unfortunately patients cascade from the learning curve of experience as doctors gain expertise. Experience and expertise improves outcomes, specialist centres and experienced doctors get the best results, but unfortunately there is no short circuiting the path to excellence, and some patients die as the doctors learn how to recognise and deal with drug toxicity.

"I've got it professor … any tummy pain and I'm to stop the pill and go straight to Casualty."

The professor smiled. He liked the formality with which Rick addressed him. He hated people calling him by his first name before he'd taken off his hat. He didn't call his patients by their first names. He showed respect so why didn't they do the same.

'Goodness what is the world like?' he mused,

'Bring back the Ernests and the Alberts.'

The Alberts and Ernests, were, according to the professor's way of thinking, a fine species of patient; a deferential species that brought him bottles at Christmas and brought the nurses chocolates at almost any time.

And Rick and Rachel noticing that their professor was on holiday in Dreamland thought it time to say goodbye and thanked him for his help on getting the drug for them.

'What nice people, I do hope he does …'

The treatment went well for Rick, and over the next four weeks he had no tummy pain and no internal bleeding. The only thing that he noticed was generalised dryness of his skin, a dryness which coalesced over his cheeks into redness and spots.

"Rick … you're going through puberty again!" giggled Rachel.

"Hope not." said Rick.

"That was worse than having cancer."

But the professor reviewing Rick in clinic was delighted with his patient's spots and this delight caused Rick and Rachel some bemusement which they assigned to the professor's eccentricity catalogue until he exclaimed,

"It means that you may be getting better."

… And he explained.

The changes in your skin mean that your skin cells have a receptor that's attracting the treatment. The sunitinib is homing in to your skin. And since it's homing in to your skin it's likely that the same receptor is also present on your tumour and that … it's also homing in on your tumour. And so with a bit of luck you should be getting better.

"Yippee!" whooped Rachel.

"Now you mustn't get too excited. You'll have to wait for the results of the scan."

A further month passed and Rick had another scan. The professor and his colleagues reviewed Rick's new scan and could see that the tumour had shrunk.

It was time for the professor's secretary to make a happy call. The professor and his secretary didn't like keeping patients waiting until their clinic appointments for good news.

Rick and Rachel were in clinic again. Most of their lives it seemed to them were spent in clinic.

"So what happens now?"

"We keep going."

Rick noticed the use of the plural form, but he was an English teacher, so it was part of the art of his own job description to notice language just as it is the doctor's job to notice abnormal clinical signs, reading disease in the faces of his patients. Rick was rather pleased with the ownership expressed by the use of the plural form. The reason that the professor liked to use the plural form, was that he felt that it gave confidence to his patients, making them feel that they were all on the same side, that they were in it together.

Christmas came and the professor noticed that Rachel seemed to be putting on weight. He kept rather quiet about the weight gain. There was a differential diagnosis when fecund females become plump. He hadn't forgotten asking a large, square sided nurse of battleship dimensions whether she was pregnant and had been mortified by her response which was,

'No, I'm just fat.'

So it had become professorial policy never to enquire if a woman was pregnant.

But then …

"We are pregnant professor. It's early days so we are keeping it quiet."

And there and then a challenge began and the challenge was to keep Rick going until the baby came. It was a point of honour for the professor. He would be dammed if he didn't get Rick there.

But there was a little problem. Just a little problem. And the problem was that Rick had become poorly again, he'd lost weight, developed tummy pain and his poor pale cheeks seemed to be hanging from his cheekbones. It was time for another scan and the professor's secretary would be unlikely to be calling Rick and Rachel with good news.

'I hate doing this.' the professor thought as he sat in the clinic consulting room facing Rick and Rachel.

'They are so nice. Can't there be good news just for once?'

"The thing is … that the trouble in your tum …"

The professor didn't like using the word cancer, it seemed just too much.

"… is just a little bit worse. Nothing too horrible but I do think that it's time for us to be thinking about another treatment for your condition."

Rachel sat forward on her chair, anxious, concern showing on her face. She was clearly pregnant now, her months showing as she counted down the time to her due day.

"There are other treatments that are available for kidney cancers … mind you we'll have to go through the same old process again of application to the PCT. But I am sure that we'll get through this again."

"What's the new drug called?"

"Temsirolimus."

"How does it work?"

"It's a little like sunitinib in that it has a similar cellular effect. There is a gene that's important in renal cell cancer called mTOR. MTOR is important in the control of cell division and its activity leads to the production of factors involved in cell oxygen content and indirectly, to the manufacture of the cell's surface receptors for blood vessels. MTOR can be inhibited by temsirolimus and this leads to patients with kidney cancer getting better! It's given intravenously and does have side effects some of which are similar to those of sunitinib.

"Tell you what, if you'd like me to do so I will introduce you to a lady who is having the drug and she can tell you about her experiences with treatment. Would you like an introduction?"

"Yes please." said Rick

"And by the way professor, what do you think of this?"

Rick lifted up his shirt to show the professor some lumps that had appeared under his skin, just over his bottom.

The professor leaned forward in his chair and peered at the lumps. His heart sank. He knew what they were, they were metastases ... areas under the skin where the cancer had spread and grown. Rick's skin bulged with deposits of cancer that distorted the tissues. These deposits were always seen as a 'Pre-terminal event'.

Medicine is full of names and labels. By giving names to symptoms and signs, by labelling horrible things, the naming process itself takes away some of the horror of the disease, naming and labelling sanitized desperation and misery, suffering and devastation. 'Subcutaneous metastases' somehow didn't seem as ghastly as 'The cancer has spread to the skin', which conjured images of 'The Alien' and poor Sigourney Weaver's skin's writhing infestation by space monsters. And 'Pre-terminal event', makes less dreadful the nastiness of the observation that in a little while, nice Rick was bound to be nice dead Rick.

But this sanitisation process clearly only functions in medical staff. These clinical labels make it easier for the doctors; there is less emotion around the formal description of horrifying symptoms and signs. But for the patients perhaps, the grimness and sterility, the stark play of the words of the clinical label is more emotive than any lay term or description.

So Rick went with Rachel into the Cancer Centre's Day Ward where he met Mrs Patel, who was sat in a very smart pink plastic recliner receiving an infusion of Temsirolimus. The Day Ward is the area of the hospital where people receive treatments such as chemotherapy and blood transfusion, treatments that do not require them to be in-patients and stay in the wards overnight. Mrs Patel was pleased to see Rick and even more pleased to chat. There's nothing like finding someone in the same black hulled boat as you are to make a situation better. Rick and Mrs Patel, pig tail and sari sat all in a row, with Rachel at 20 weeks pregnant, looking on.

"I've heard the heartbeat professor."

"I bet it's a boy." said the professor.

"How did you know that?"

"We have our ways."

There is talk of a very successful gynaecologist who always knew the sex of the unborn. Apparently he'd say

"It's going to be a girl!"

… Whilst writing in the records,

"Boy."

Of course when the baby was born if he was 'Right,' his prediction would be greeted by confirmation of the view that the doctor is all seeing, but if told he was 'Wrong,' he would merely indicate with a tap of his fountain pen the place in his notes where he'd written the sex of the child and state that the mother had remembered his prediction incorrectly.

You see doctors always do have to be right.

So the professor battled with the PCT over the prescription of temsirolimus and this time, unlike the situation with sunitinib, there was no struggle and he won through without a fight.

'What a pity,' the professor thought,

'I do like a bit of a struggle!'

But he was joking about the struggle. He hated conflict. The professor abhorred confrontation.

In cancer medicine, treatment with a new drug is usually preceded by an assessment scan. Treatment is then started and at the end of about two months of the new medication the scans are repeated to assess whether or not there has been a response. The two month interval is chosen because it is generally sufficient to have given the treatment a chance of working. The doctors look at the new scan and compare the abnormalities seen on the new scan with the pre-treatment changes. If the scan shows that the tumour has shrunk then it's champagne all round and the treatment continues. If the tumour is bigger, then the treatment is stopped because there is objective evidence of treatment failure and it's straight to the brandy butt.

When the doctors look at scans of cancer patients, they study the images and attempt to define the extent of the cancer. The normal structures are viewed and the radiologist asks himself whether the organs are in the right place and have the right shape. He will then look at individual organs such as the liver or lungs and assess the significance of the dots and spots that he might see within the organ's substance. If the liver has a non-uniform appearance then computer image contrast controls are adjusted to evaluate the density of the little spots in the liver. By this means he can work out from density measurements whether the spots seen in the liver are due to spread of the cancer or to non-malignant cysts. Then the radiologist goes on to peer at the lymph nodes and measure their dimensions. If their diameter is beyond normal limits, the change in size of the nodes may be because of the spread of cancer to those nodes, but not necessarily, because in the end all that one looks at on a scan are shadows. Shadows aren't pathology and shape is not diagnostic. However from the shapes and shadows conclusions are formed of the extent and dimensions of the tumour.

The radiologist, Dr Hoff, sat with the professor at a bank of computer screens, flicked through the CT scan images of Rick's abdomen and stroked his moustache. It wasn't the professor's moustache that Dr Hoff stroked, but not through a lack of desire on Dr Hoff's part. Hunched together in the dimmed light of the X-ray reporting room, Dr Hoff scrolled down through the cross sectional images, pointing out to the professor the various landmarks of the structures in Rick's abdomen and pelvis, with a,

"Harrumph ..."

... followed by a naming of an organ and an audible exclamation mark.

"Harrumph ... spleen!"

Together they could see the precise size of the tumour in Rick's abdomen... an absolutely huge mass extending out from the kidney. And viewing Rick's spine ... what had previously seemed like mongoose bites had become the imprints of the ravenous jaws of a howling tiger. The radiologist using computer software put a cursor over the tumour and measured its diameter. The tumour spanned 20 centimetres in its maximal dimension. It was enormous. The radiologist shook his head, and murmured,

"Poor chap."

At which the professor said,

"Yup!"

Which pretty much summed things up.

Rick started treatment with temsirolimus attending the Day Ward each week for his hourly infusion. He became anaemic after about one months' treatment. Anaemia is common in cancer patients and has many causes. Anaemia may be due to vitamin or iron deficiency as in a patient without cancer, or it may be due to blood loss, for example from bleeding of the kidney tumour into the urinary tract. Much more commonly it can be caused by an effect of the cancer itself. The presence of the cancer inhibits the production of red blood cells by the patient's own bone marrow, and it does so because the cancer secretes chemicals into its host's blood stream.

Rick had become a little breathless and very tired and these are symptoms of anaemia. The treatment of anaemia in cancer patients is by blood transfusion, because patients are unlikely to be made better by any other means. Blood is given, and within a few days of the transfusion the patient's symptoms ease. And so it was with Rick.

Meanwhile the weeks passed and Rachel was entering the late stages of her pregnancy.

"Look!" she said,

"Those little bumps under Rick's skin, they seem to be smaller."

The professor inspected Rick's skin and yes the lumps certainly had shrunk. It was time for a re-assessment scan. The professor was a bit worried about what the scan would show. He was worried because Rick had developed high blood levels of calcium, found by routine blood testing.

In cancer patients, high blood calcium can be due to spread of cancer to bone. This is a situation where cancer cells are borne by the blood stream to settle in bone. There, lodged in the fabric of the bone, the cancer cells grow and divide and eat away at the bone matrix. As they grow, the cancer cells spit out calcium from the bone into the blood stream. There is another reason for a raised blood calcium level. High calcium can be caused by the release from the tumour itself of a hormone that interferes with the normal regulation of blood calcium levels. The regulatory controls are reset, and lead to an increase in the activity of cells in bone called osteoclasts. In turn, these osteoclast cells are stimulated to dissolve bone and the bones' calcium content is released from the bone into the blood so that blood calcium levels become unnaturally high.

This high calcium level may lead to a galaxy of strange symptoms ranging from confusion to constipation. This is because high blood calcium levels bathing the bodies' tissues interfere with the way that the bodies' cells conduct electrical currents. By doing so, high calcium induces a state of near paralysis in some body structures and the gut becomes immobile and it gets to be difficult to think.

So it's important to treat raised blood calcium levels.

But unfortunately this situation is a near terminal event, the second near terminal event for Rick. The median survival of a cancer patient with high calcium levels is in the order of two to three months. And Rachel was 30 weeks pregnant. It would be touch and go.

The professor, the nurses and the junior doctors in the Oncology Department all knew about Rachel and Rick. Rick and Rachel had conducted themselves with dignity and grace, never complaining always cheerful. The professor felt inherently that they were both fully aware of the outcome … they understood that time was very limited, and that they didn't want to discuss that outcome with him. They didn't want to confront the thought of death, wanted to manage a day at a time.

And there was objective evidence that this was their view. In the course of Rick's illness he had filled in a questionnaire that had been designed by the doctors to assess how patients dealt with their illnesses. The questionnaire probed their feelings on a broad range of issues from diagnosis to diet, from life quality to the quality of the treatment that they were given. Rick, in filling in the questionnaire, had written that he didn't really want to know about the prognosis that he faced but would rather get on from day to day and trust in the medical staff to let him know if his situation looked like it was deteriorating. He'd also written that he knew that he was going to die and that he had come to terms with that prospect, understanding that everything that could be done had been done and that the medical and nursing teams looking after him had given him all that they could do. He knew, as he wrote in the questionnaire, that

'... In the end it was just one of those things.'

The professor had seen his comments. The comments had stopped him from breathing for about ten minutes.

Doctors are counselled that when they are about to discuss issues such as death with their patients, to first take a view from their patients as to how they feel about their situation before blundering into a painful statement about life expectancy. The professor thought that it was time to make sure that Rick and Rachel understood the seriousness of their situation and he began tentatively to explore their need to define prognosis.

"Rick, how do you think you are getting on?"

"Well professor, I think that things aren't so good ..."

Rick peered at the professor through his rectangular steel framed glasses and the magnification made his eyes seem distant and distracted.

"Yes Rick. I am sorry."

The professor was sorry. He felt for Rick and Rachel. The couple had somehow by-passed his defences. He really, really, really, wished with all his heart that he could get Rick better.

'Bloody cancer. What a bugger.'

"Would you like me to tell you anything else about your situation?"

"I don't think so professor. I am OK."

Rachel edged forward on her seat. Her face flushed, and her eyes reddened.

Rick paused and turned to his wife.

"Is there anything that you would like to know Rachel?"

Rachel seemed to draw on a reservoir of enormous emotional strength the size of the Pacific, gathered herself together, took a big breath and said,

"No Rick, I'm OK. We'll talk about it later at home and if there is anything that we want to discuss, we'll ask the professor, won't we?"

So the professor knew that Rick knew and Rachel knew.
And Rachel knew that Rick knew and the professor knew.
And Rick knew that the professor knew and that Rachel
knew. So why should they talk about IT any further? There
was no point. There was so much that was understood and so
much that didn't need confronting. Neither Rachel nor Rick
nor the professor really wanted to talk about the time that
Rick had left. And … why should they talk? There was no
gain. Slap the facts in a big hessian bag, weigh it down with
granite cobblestones, whirl the bag around your head and
toss the bag in a river. We all find our way.

But what they did want to know, or rather who, they did
want to know was a certain little one who was growing in
Rachel's belly, the swimmer in a not so secret sea, unfurling,
coiling and curling in the paddling pool of Rachel's womb. And
the pregnancy was becoming more and more obvious. Day by
day, week by week, the unborn child was getting bigger.

But as the baby got bigger so did poor Rick get smaller,
the weight falling from his rag and bone frame. Weight loss is
one of the symptoms that cancer patients hate almost more
than pain. The thinness of a cancer patient brands them, stig-
matises them, makes them stand out from other men and
women in the check out queue at Sainsbury's. Rick's cheek
bones would have won prizes at Belsen and his buttocks were
lollipops on sticks.

It was time for another scan. The radiologist compared what
had been seen in Rick's abdomen on his old scans to what could
be seen on his current scan. And it was clear that things were
much worse. The tumour that had measured 20cm in maximal
diameter now measured 30cm and as to Rick's spine …

"Looks like the patient's spine is held together by tumour!
If it weren't for the cancer there would be nothing of him!"
commented Dr Hoff wryly.

"Hmmm …" mumbled the professor,

"Poor chap."

So it was bad news time again.

"But look …" said Rachel,

"The skin lumps are smaller."

Rick pulled up his shirt and the professor could see that Rachel was right. The lumps had halved in size. This is a state which is described by oncologists as a 'mixed response', where part of the tumour shrinks usually as a result of treatment and part of the tumour grows despite treatment. In this situation the cancer doctor has to make a decision whether or not to continue treatment or change the drugs. The decision is based on the bottom line for the patient. The treating clinician has to decide whether on balance the patient is better or worse off as a result of his current treatment? If the balance is viewed as being positive then the treatment is continued, but if the balance is negative, then …

In the case of Rick, the situation was a close judgment call. The professor explained,

"Look it is clear that parts of your tumour … the bits under the skin are responding but other parts aren't doing so well. So I think that what we should is continue the temsirolimus but also add another drug. What do you think?"

Rick nodded and commented,

"Seems logical professor. I would go for that."

The options were limited. Rick had almost come to the end of the treatment road, the place on the map where the tarmac extends to the edge of the cliff. But through all of this he was still going to work, on public transport, to his beloved class of adoring six formers.

Rachel was at 36 weeks.

The doctors would need to extend the edge of the cliff.

"So the next treatment is called interferon. It's given by injection under the skin three times a week. We have had this treatment available for almost 30 years. The side effects are usually just mild flu like symptoms that come on an hour or so after the injection, and then last a couple of hours. These side effects can usually be made easier by giving two paracetamol tablets before the injection. Another thing that can be helpful is having the injection last thing at night … if you do this then with any luck you should be able to sleep through the side effects."

Rachel had been trained as a nurse and she volunteered to give the injections.

"It's a chance to get my own back professor … no honestly Rick I'm only joking!"

Interferon had been known about for many years. It is one of a group of chemicals made by the body's white blood cells that are part of a complex defence system that acts to tone up the body to enable it to fight infection. In the early 1980s the manufacturing process for interferon had been worked out and interferon became available as a potential new treatment for any number of medical conditions where it was considered that a slack and rusty immune system needed a bit of spit and polish.

The rationale for interferon having any effect in cancer was based on the findings that cancer patients had lowered immunity and that people who had over active immune systems which had caused illnesses such as asthma and eczema had a decreased chance of developing some cancers. And so it was hoped that interferon could be used as a drug that could treat patients with cancer. The idea was that interferon would energise the patients' paralysed immune system and the re-energised bodies' natural processes would then march on and be able to reject tumours.

So as soon as interferon became available commercially, one of the major cancer charities cornered the market in interferon and announcements were made that the Charity would use interferon to begin a war against cancer. Cynics said that the main reason that the Charity was doing this was to increase its appeal in the competitive fundraising market, not because of any real hope that interferon would work.

Battle metaphors are broadly employed in the struggle against cancer, and the Charity was recapitulating Richard Nixon's 1975 clarion call of 'A war against cancer'.

In the 1980s interferon was used to treat patients with many different types of cancer. Trials of interferon took place in people with leukaemia and lymphoma, lung cancer and bowel cancer together with many other tumour types. Doctors treated patients hoping to see their tumours respond, but there were very few patients who improved with treatment. The campaign generals met and considered that overall interferon was not the magic bullet that would cure all cancer. The cancer charity's crusade was unfortunately lost, but on the way to defeat the troops achieved some spectacular individual victories. Amongst the campaign triumphs was the battle against kidney cancer. Patients with kidney cancer responded to interferon. The response rates were low, and the time for which patients got better was measured in months rather than decades, but some months were a whole lot better than no months: the responses were significant.

Rachel had reached 38 weeks.

Rick needed to be seen more regularly and was coming up to Clinic weekly. Rick became anaemic again and needed a blood transfusion. He sat calmly in the Day Ward blood tipping in through a drip, a small pile of books and the Guardian for company, bemused almost, by the procession of events around him, the parade of doctors and nurses, the patients in treatment, the wheelchairs and chocolates. Rachel as ever, ever present, watching over him, loving Rick.

Rick's legs and belly became swollen. He wore size 56" waist trousers tacked to his shoulders by braces, narrow torso suspended over the lower body of a larger man.

"What's this due to professor?"

So the professor explained that there are many causes of the swelling. But it was likely that the cause in Rick was pressure of the tumour on the great vessels inside his belly. The compression of the veins and lymph vessels stopped blood returning to the heart and so his legs and belly had swollen to contain the fluid.

Rick nodded.

"So does that mean that the tumour has grown?"

"Yes Rick …"

This was the first time that the professor had addressed Rick using his first name.

Rick nodded again. Nodded just once. Rick understood. The professor understood that Rick had understood.

No more needed to be said. They had communicated. And Rachel watched over the words.

Rachel was at 40 weeks.

"They're bringing me in professor. They're going to induce me next week. We are making arrangements for Rick to come in too so that we can be together."

It was ward round time and the trail of doctors and medical students trooped along to the ward adjoining the Labour Ward where Rick was ensconced. He'd been admitted unwell from home, quite breathless and more swollen. He was in a single bedded room, a luxury for NHS patients!

Rachel stood at the bottom of his bed, in dressing gown and nightie, arms folded over her belly, anxious, waiting for us, and waiting for delivery.

Rick, breathless and swollen looked up at the medical team.

"We've decided, professor that I won't come in to see the Caesarean." he panted.

"No." said Rachel,

"Rick will wait here and his sister will keep me company."

The professor looked at Rick, looked with a level of anxiety and concern. He noticed that Rick was breathing at a rate that was twice the normal rate and that his colour wasn't good. Rick had a blue tinge to his lips, which told the medical team that the levels of oxygen in Rick's blood had fallen far below a healthy level needed to sustain life.

The professor turned to the junior doctors.

"What's his sats?"

This was code for oxygen saturation, an indicator of how well Rick's lungs were working in providing oxygen to his red blood cells.

"59%."

Rachel became tenser. She stroked her belly for comfort.

"Any cause for the sats?"

"Perhaps we should go and look through the blood results and X-rays, Prof?"

This, from the excellent and very serious registrar, whose job it was mostly to keep the professor and any other stray consultants under control. The registrar needed to discuss Rick's management out of earshot of Rick and Rachel.

The doctors, serious, sombre, gathered in the ward office, grouped around the computer screens. The registrar searched the computerised X-ray index for Rick's chest X-ray and displayed it on the screen. Rick's X-ray was a ghastly battlefield of all that could be wrong in the lungs. A spray of white pellets and marbles, ping pong and tennis balls decorated Rick's lung fields, the shadows of fluid pools filled the corners of his lungs, filled the fissures that separated the lobes of his lungs and drenched his lymph channels. This was a picture that could be seen in late stage cancer where there has been extensive spread to the lungs. Rick's heart was enlarged with the effort of pumping blood through the morass of tumour secondary's that cluttered his lungs. It was a wonder that Rick could breathe at all.

The doctors seemed collectively to suck in breath and shake heads.

"We've got to get him through," said the professor.

"Rick's to have everything."

The medical team re-grouped in Rick's room.

"A little bit of bother there Rick. We'll get it sorted."

The professor glanced at Rachel whose eyes welled and reddened. She looked away. The level of pathos in the room had reached saturation and it seemed as though even the professor was about to cry. A couple of the juniors left the room. They were crying too.

"So when are you being done Rachel?"

"They are coming for me in about 30 minutes professor."

"Best of luck."

"I'll be all right!"

The professor turned to the juniors.

"Steroids please … antibiotics and anticoagulants. OK?"

The drugs were written up.

"And oxygen."

On his way home that evening the professor looked in to Rick's room. Rick was sitting up in bed with an oxygen mask on. His close family were gathered around the bed, brother and sister-in-law. At the bottom of the bed in a white crib lay the new family member. A beautiful boy, fine featured, at peace, sleeping quietly. Babies born by Caesarean section have none of the tissue swelling that comes with vaginal delivery and are particularly lovely. But this was a particularly lovely Caesarean child … it wasn't just the style of birth that had produced the handsome baby.

The professor worried about Rick on his way home from work, at home whilst making supper, worried about Rick when he was having his shower and worried about him again when he lay down to sleep.

"What's the matter darling?"

And the professor told his wife.

"You have done all that you could sweetheart."

"But it's not enough."

She held him close and stroked his back.

"I know …"

Morning came and the professor went to Rick's room on his way before going to his office. His approach to the ward was tentative, not wishing to confront the possibility of Rick's death.

Rick was sat up in bed on plumped up pillows. His head, neck and the upper parts of his shoulders were inserted into a cubical clear plastic hood the size of an old fashioned hair drier. This type of hood is used to deliver high concentrations of oxygen, higher levels than could come through a face mask.

Rick stared out at the professor, peered through steamed up glasses, peered through plumes of swirling clouds of gas and moisture droplets, peered through the crumpled plastic of his oxygen hood. Rick smiled and nodded a morning's welcome to his professor. Rick's breathing was rapid and shallow. His skin had become mottled and blue. His belly was hugely distended and his legs enormously swollen.

The baby had been moved out of the crib and was lying at the foot of Rick's bed. Rick wasn't touching the baby. The family remained gathered around Rick's bed. They hadn't gone home.

"How are you Rick?"

"I'm all right ..." Rick gasped.

" ... It doesn't really matter," he panted, sweat staining his pyjamas, glasses steaming up with the effort of breathing.

The professor wondered whether Rick was commenting about the meaninglessness of his own life in the context of the span of infinite humanity, and it maybe was that he was talking about just that.

"Are you comfortable Rick?"

"I'm OK. Really, I'm quite OK."

The fingers of Rick's right hand lifted from the sheets.

The professor turned to the sound of a door opening and to Rachel in fluffy slippers and towelling dressing gown, coming into the room, her face puffy with crying. She came over to Rick's bed and took his hand. Rachel looked up from Rick's face and smiled at the professor.

"We're all right. Honestly."

"See you later ..."

It was Friday afternoon and the medical and nursing teams had gathered again to discuss Rick's management over the weekend. There was not the usual chatter and frivolity. The doctors and nurses were quiet, grim, distressed, focussed. They liked Rick; they liked his tranquillity, admired his braveness, were amazed at his calmness, and felt deeply the tragedy of his situation.

The professor tried to draw the teams together to define Rick's care over the weekend. In the doctor's office, they pondered again the awfulness of the chest X-rays and as indicated by the blood tests, the serial daily deteriorations in Rick's kidney and liver function. They wondered about changing antibiotics, they speculated about adding yet more diuretics, they considered trying antifungals, they discussed adding inotropes, and they thought about obtaining yet more specialist consultations from colleagues in other disciplines.

And then in a moment of hesitation, the intensity of their concentration was broken by a small and quiet voice.

"He's dying," said Louise the Macmillan nurse.

And her statement smacked at the doctors and nurses, shocked them, stopped them, for although they knew that Rick was dying, they had not come to terms with the prospect of his death and the reality of what dying meant in the context of Rick and them. They wanted Rick to live, they wanted him better, they wanted Rick to be playing with his kid, they wanted him to see the kid grow, they wanted him to see his child have his own children. For in some way Rick's specialness had taken their hearts. Cruel fate had to be good fate just this once. Fate, be good, please don't let Rick die.

"I think that we should make him comfortable," Louise continued.

This is a euphemism for 'It's time to give him some morphine and give up on the medical heroics.'

"Let's go and see him, and we'll …"

The professor's voice trailed away in to stuttering silence.

The ward round swayed through the corridors to Rick's bedside. The hood was off.

"I couldn't hack it professor," Rick wheezed, the effort of speaking too much for him. Rachel became Rick's voice.

"It was too uncomfortable. He felt claustrophobic. He took it off."

Rick's head slumped, and his chin rested on his chest.

Rick's was breathing at a rate of 60 breaths a minute. The normal rate is 13 or so breaths each minute.

Rick's skin had become mottled, showing the changes seen when a person is near to death, the changes that occur when the heart fails in its efforts to provide an adequate circulation.

Rick's belly was swollen and his legs had become elephantine. His toes had blackened, dire signs of a collapsed circulation.

Rick's brother and sister were crying quietly.

Rick's baby was lying sleeping between Rick's legs.

The professor came close to Rachel and whispered,

"Could we have a chat Rachel?"

Back in the doctors' office, Rachel and the professor spoke in the presence of the Macmillan nurse.

"We are going to carry on with all of the treatment. Nothing will be stopped. Every effort will continue to be made for Rick. I don't think he is comfortable though. What do you think Rachel?"

"I agree, he is distressed by the effort of having to breathe at such a rate."

Rachel's tone had become professionalised. It was the nurse in her taking over …

"We'd like to give him just a small dose of morphine. It won't hasten … things … but it will ensure that his mind is at rest and that he's less distressed by having to breathe so rapidly."

"I agree professor. He needs to be made comfortable."

"Would you like to add anything Louise?"

"… Rick mustn't be allowed to suffer. That's our priority at this point."

"Would you like to ask anything Rachel?"

"No. Thanks. I think I understand."

They stood up and walked from the office, Louise to arrange for the morphine to be given, Rachel to return to Rick and her family, the professor to his own office, and all to puzzle over the cruelty of fickle fate.

At the very end of the afternoon, at going home time the professor returned to the ward. It was 6.30 pm and Louise was there too.

"Shall we look in?"

They peeped around the door frame, to the huddled mass, of family, baby and Rick. The family in mourning, Rick unconscious and near death, the baby sleeping quietly.

"Can I help at all? Is there anything that I can do?"

The professor was conscious of the inadequacy of his words.

Rachel brought her right hand to her mouth and shook her head.

"I will be available over the weekend."

And the professor shuffled out backwards from Rick's room, and felt like shuffling backwards all the way home.

On Monday morning the professor bumped into Louise as he came into the hospital.

"He was such a nice man."

"He woke up and asked for cup of tea yesterday afternoon."

"WHAT!"

"Hadn't you heard?

"... He had a cup of tea!"

"Chriiiisssssssssssssssssst!

"You are joking?"

"Nope. It's a miracle. He's recovered."

"What? I cannot believe that. Recovered? He was 99% dead on Friday afternoon. It's impossible."

"Go and have a look for yourself then."

So the professor went to Rick's room and saw for himself the miracle on Hope Reigns Eternal Ward.

Rick was sitting up in bed, holding the baby.

Rick wasn't breathless. He was breathing normally.

Rick's ante-mortem skin staining had gone.

Rick looked fine.

The family were there, brother and sister and sister in law. And they were smiling.

"How are you professor?" asked Rick.

"I'm fine thanks Rick. How are you?"

"Good."

"Looks like you'll be going home shortly."

"Really professor? I'd like that."

Rick and Rachel and the baby went home on Wednesday morning. Arrangements made in double quick time. Against all odds, snatched from death, as near to death as never been seen before to recover. A miracle. Rick's big adventure.

Rick had some time with his son, precious time to hold his child, precious time for Rachel to hold them both, but then in love and with peace, time had its way.

Chapter 2
All My Trials

"So, how did it all begin?"

… You ask … how it all began?

I remember how it started … *how could I ever forget*?

It was exactly two years ago. Two years ago to the day. The 2nd of June. I was in the shower.

Water on.

I can see the bar of soap … there it is.

I have scorched into my memory the image of the bar of soap grasped in my right hand and pushed into my left armpit. The image of the soap seems to me to this day to carry with it around its edges sinister fluorescence, bubbling bursts of violent flames. And as it moved into my armpit the soap bumped up against this … thing.

And I froze.

And I looked down. Raised my arm.

There it was.

The thing.

In my armpit, there in my left armpit.

It was the size of a golf ball. Hard and round.

And I whispered,

"Fuck it"

I should have shouted,

"FUCK it!"

It would have been a more appropriate response.

I sensed immediately that the lump was a very big deal.

I just knew that something completely horrible was up.

J. Waxman, *The Elephant in the Room*,
DOI 10.1007/978-0-85729-895-9_2,
© Springer-Verlag London Limited, 2012

I felt sick. My hands shook. My heart raced. I was scared shitless … I just … well … I just … absolutely panicked. An army of ants rampaged in my guts.

And the lump throbbed.

It seemed to be telling me that it was important.

Golf ball, wish it had been a golf ball.

So my next thought after the fuck it thought, was the what to do thought. But the what to do next thought got muddled and forgotten and I dropped the soap. I felt in my right arm-pit. There was nothing there. Shower still on, I passed my hands over the rest of my body looking for anything strange, anything unusual. But there was nothing else alien to be felt. I washed off the bubbles and got out of the shower.

And then I remembered the what to do next thought.

And the answer was pretty straight forward and that was to go to my GP.

I didn't bother phoning the surgery. Would have been just told that I could have an appointment in ten days time. I didn't do ten days. I have always done now. So I went there … it's my way just to do things, just to get on.

I didn't go to work … just went straight down the road and into the GP's surgery. I remember almost in freeze frame, pushing open the door to silence. It was as if the volume control had been switched right off. And then the sound came back again arising in a big bubble that welled from a small crowd of shrieking kids and fretful mums. I went straight to the reception desk … which was more of a keep away barrier than a desk.

The receptionist peeped over a stack of patient notes and stared at me peeking out from between the ferns,

"Have you an appointment?" she asked.

And I said,

"No!"

She peered over her half moons at me as if I was the fly in her soup, glanced at her computer screen as if she was the original model for the drag queen bank clerk in Little Britain and said,

"Not sure if doctor will see you without an appointment".

And so I told her that I thought he would, as I was very worried that I might have a very serious problem.

"I'll wait until he has a space to see me," I said.

Not waiting for her reply, I sat down and waded through the curly cornered copies of *Hello* magazine, with a nonchalance that said that I could wait all day if necessary and I am not going until you sort me out, whilst the legions of fully armed panic continued to have their way with my flesh. I was brazening it out with that gorgon receptionist and I wasn't going to look up from the marriage of Gavin and Colleen to give her the satisfaction of a chance to tell me that the doctor wouldn't see me.

After an hour's wait, at the end of the morning's list, the doctor came out of his clinic room. I watched him as he walked along the corridor and he saw me staring at him. He came into the waiting room, smiled a hello and said,

"We don't usually have the pleasure of your company at the surgery, why not come in and have a chat?"

My doctor is a little chap with glinting John Lennon glasses and one of those droopy moustaches that were in fashion in the late 60s. He's very decent and I bet he's the sort that doesn't send his kids to private school even though he can afford it.

So I followed him into his room for a chat.

Chat? Hardly! It wasn't about girls, the football or my Beemer! He asked me what was wrong and then examined me. I showed him the 'thing', pinching it between my fingers, and he felt it too, pushing at it with his finger tips. He became quiet, seemed to think for a bit and then he told me as I got dressed, that he thought that the lump was a lymph node, the sort of thing that lay people call 'glands'. Then he explained that glands like the one that I had in my armpit can come up when there is infection, but from the look of him when he said the word,

'Infection.'

I knew that there was no chance that he really thought that the gland was due to an infection. But what he did say was that the node was there and shouldn't be there.

Then pausing for a moment he tipped his glasses up the slope of his nose with his finger, scratched his head and then asked me some very strange questions. Well they were strange to me then, but nowadays, they are not strange at all, they are most familiar. Almost every doctor asks me the same questions. I have had the questions so often repeated that they are almost friends.

He asked me if I had had any night sweats, temperatures, or had lost any weight or had alcohol related pain or skin itching.

The answer was 'No' to all of his questions.

Nowadays I understand why it is that the doctors ask me these questions ... it's to find out if I have any specific symptoms caused by my tumour. You see the tumour makes peculiar chemicals that cause fevers and weight loss ... how weird is that then?

"Look," he said when he had finished with his probing.

"I think we better get you seen at the hospital. The 'thing', as you call it, in your armpit, well, it's a lymph node, as I have said and in my opinion it shouldn't be there. So if it's OK with you I am going to refer you to a surgeon.

"I should warn you, though warn is probably the wrong word, that the surgeon will want to take it out.

"I'd like to get you sorted out, so I'll fax a letter to the surgeon today and you should get seen within the next couple of weeks."

Then he paused again. I think that my GP specialised in pauses.

"Tell you what ... I'll phone him now and see if we can get you seen as soon as possible. If you'd like to wait outside whilst I give him a ring please?"

Not that I did like waiting outside, it felt as though I was being dismissed, not allowed to hear the real truth about my lump, a truth that the big boys were party to, but I was not. I wanted to know what they really thought about me!

I shuffled off whilst he made the call. It was back to the magazines in the waiting room. Not for very long though, not long enough to get to the bottom of the Gavin and Colleen affair. But come to think of it, even though I did feel excluded from the medical chat, I don't think that I was in any state to hear any horrible words at the time. I realise that it was actually very good of him to make the call. Very good indeed.

So my appointment to see the surgeon was issued for the next day. The fact that the appointment had been issued so promptly worried me more than a little. But at least I was getting sorted out quickly.

I went by myself to the hospital, had neither friend nor lover to keep me company. I wished that I had someone to talk to, someone to remind me of what had been said, someone to give just a little comfort. Wished I had someone. On and off it's been a lonely business this illness. And life had been so good up to then, great job, great flat ... too busy though with the work, hence ... the ... you know ... lack of friends.

I say on and off a lonely business. Funny thing is that it's not lonely in the hospital; it's almost fun being sick and in hospital. How bizarre is that ... but when you think about it, maybe it's not so bonkers, because in hospital you are cared for and safe. And that's the paradox, because even though you might be mortally sick there's the camaraderie and community, there's always someone to ask how you are and share your troubles, always a whole bunch of people fighting for you trying to get you better.

The surgeon was brilliant though, brisk, as they are, and to the point as they are ... He said,

"We could mess around sticking needles in, trying to get a core biopsy ..."

And I had no idea what he meant by a core biopsy so I just nodded,

"It will save a lot of time if we just take it out. We'll get the answer without faffing around. It'll be a day case. You won't need to stay in. Any questions?"

The way that the surgeon put things made it all seem very simple and I really didn't have any questions.

So the next day they injected some local anaesthetic in my armpit and cut the lump out. Not much waiting around, sorted, I thought. I thought that it was all over then because they didn't issue me with any outpatient appointment for review. I assumed that was it. All over and carry on as though nothing at all had happened or could happen. Silly, silly, innocent little me. They did tell me to go to my GP to get the stitches taken out, so when the nurse was doing just that in the GP's surgery, she asked me just by way of conversation, when I was going back to see them again.

"What, no appointment?"

She soon got me an appointment for the hospital for review.

So it was the surgeons again.

"We've got good news for you. It's all out and we're going to refer you to an oncologist."

I asked them what it was that they had got out.

"Oh it was a lymphoma, nothing to worry about. Professor Andrews will tell you everything that you need to know. It'll all be sorted out. Don't worry at all."

I can still hear those words echoing down the years … Don't worry at all.

Mind you if I had any sense I would have followed their advice. You see there really wasn't any point in worrying at all. Worrying really doesn't help.

Professor Andrews. What a professor he was. Wherever he was there was noise. Red faced. Blustering. Pin stripe double breasted suit. Posh.

The nurse showed me into his room. He was sitting behind a big desk. There were two medical students there. They looked badly frightened. I am sure that he terrified them. He looked up as I came into the room, stared at me as if sort of summing me up and then without any ado just said,

"You could die from this you know."

Oh the shock of it. And then,

"But I am going to do my best to see that you don't."

And then he just went straight in with the business end.

"You have got a high grade lymphoma. It's a type of cancer. Can be nasty. You are going to have to have chemotherapy. The treatment will make you feel bloody awful. It could possibly kill you. You will lose all your hair. You'll be frightfully sick. But at the end of it all you'll probably be all right … Actually."

I wasn't too sure about the actually. But I did like his bluntness and directness. I knew that he cared and was on my side. In a funny way the bombshells didn't hurt, they felt good. His words were inspirational in a weird way. It was as if he understood me and would be fighting for me. It was as though it was us against the lymphoma, him and me, not just me, alone and unsupported. He was in my team and my team was going to win.

At the time I had been going through an awful phase, I'd become angry, really cross with everyone and everything.

Why me? I'd thought.

"Now," said Professor Andrews,

"You're probably thinking, why me?"

And I thought … that man can read my mind. And he looked at me, as if he was hearing my thoughts, so I nodded. I'd been doing quite a lot of nodding at doctors.

"It's a phase you go through. If you weren't thinking that we'd be worried about you.

"It's what happens, if you are lucky. There are classical phases in the process of coming to terms with any life event of significance, phases that you go through as a patient facing profound illness. The first phase is called 'Denial'. It's when you fail to engage emotionally with the fact of illness. You carry on as though nothing at all has happened.

"The next phase that you pass through emotionally in dealing with the burden of your illness is the 'Why me' phase. You graduate to thinking about what it is that you have done in your life that has caused the lymphoma, you search for reasons …

"But let me tell you that, actually, there is nothing that you have done. It's just all down to bloody bad luck. Beastly bad luck in fact."

I said to him and I remember it well,

"That's me professor. I'm there. I'm there in the bad luck phase."

"Yup! Let me tell you …"

And Professor Andrews started to wag his finger at me.

"There's nothing, actually, that you have done wrong. There's no relationship to diet, bad behaviour … anything."

I had wondered about the bad behaviour!

"It's likely to be in the genes but what it is in the bloody genes that's caused the lymphoma we really don't know. And to tell you the truth we don't really care about that at the moment. What we do care about is getting you bloody well better."

I was amazed at his language. But it was funny; funny odd, how strange that his words and manner gave me such assurance. It was inspiring to hear him talk in such a confident way. It was wonderful.

"Anyway, the next thing that you will experience emotionally is anger. You will get bloody well cross at everybody and everything. Mind you they probably deserve it. So go for it!

"Then after that there comes acceptance. Bit hippy'ish that, mind you. Peace and love and all that nonsense. Some people get fixed at one stage in the process of coming to terms with illness and that's not good emotionally.

"Anyway I digress. Here's the point."

Professor Andrews' discussion about emotions seemed to be coming to an end and it was on to the real business, the practical stuff.

"You'll be needing scans and a bone marrow test. Bloody hurts the bone marrow test. So don't be a little girl about it. Take it like a man."

I would try. I wondered whether he told the girls to take it like a man?

"All right? Any questions?"

I had none. No questions at all. He waved a few forms at me and I was dismissed, off to get my CT scans, blood tests and bone marrow assessment.

The CT scans were fine. Simple really, just a lot of lying around.

Then I had to have a whole lot of special blood tests done to characterise my blood group and look for genetic changes in my white cells. They asked if I would mind giving extra blood samples for their research and I was pleased to be useful, so of course I agreed to do so but what a lot of blood they took. They made me sign my consent to having the samples taken for research. I found that odd. It was as if what they were doing in their research was somehow questionable.

It was a huge amount of blood.

"Don't worry!" the doctor said, "You've got pints of the stuff!"

Next thing for me was the bone marrow test. I had to lie down on a bed. They didn't really explain what they were doing, just told me that there would be an injection of local anaesthetic and that I would feel a pushing sensation. The local anaesthetic was injected under my skin and on the top of my pelvis … just here … over my hip at the side. I could feel the needle scrape the bone. And then the lady doctor leant on me, she leant her elbow on my thigh! And as she leaned she pushed a huge needle in to my side. The needle sank straight down on the bone. Wow … was that painful or what? Then she seemed to screw the needle into the bone turning it around and around until with a little thunk it entered the bone marrow cavity. Oh that really hurt! Just thinking of that first marrow test still makes my eyes water … and I can feel my legs cross involuntarily.

I was told later that the doctor hadn't waited long enough for the local anaesthetic to work. It's like the dentist … if the dentist waits after the injection of local, then the anaesthetic has time to have an effect and the filling is painless.

The hurt got worse. The marrow test hurt most when she said, "I am just going to draw out another sample."

Eeek.

There seemed to be a great sucking and pulling and a terrible aching, but then suddenly the test was over.

She turned away from me and fussed around with some slides, spreading out my bone marrow on the glass. She swilled out her needles and syringes into an assortment of glass bottles, smiled at me and then swooshed away. It was all over, and then it was time for me to get off the bed and limp home. The marrow test ache lingered around for days.

It was clinic time again, and I saw Professor Andrews, who told me that although the,

"Scans were clear …"

You know they always seem to start with the good news … and I know now to wait for the ends of the doctors' paragraphs.

" … the marrow is involved."

The doctors use words like 'involved' thinking that they aren't being technical but they are of course being technical and what they think is lay language, is frequently incomprehensible jargon to the lay people that they are trying to inform. The words that they consider to be simplified descriptions are almost as incomprehensible as the grossly arcane technical terms that they reserve for their own conversations.

But I got to know just exactly what 'involved' meant as soon as Professor Andrews explained that the genetic tests had shown the lymphoma cells to be in the marrow.

What did that mean to me? Well it defined my treatment path, my journey.

Professor Andrews continued with his explanation, leaning forward and staring at me as if to emphasize the point that he was about to make; it was clearly an important one for him.

"You know this is a teaching hospital don't you?"

I found this statement puzzling as it seemed an open ended observation whose relevance to me and my illness could not be discerned.

"So … it is our duty to try and advance medicine …"

I still had no idea what he was getting at.

Ah … so this is what he was getting at …

"So … as I am sure you can probably understand, at this hospital we are involved in clinical trials in which we compare a new with an older treatment, hoping to show that the new treatment is actually better than the old."

He saw that I was balking at the words 'Better than the old.' And I was doing just that, the words worried me. I wanted to have the best of all new treatments not some old fashioned rubbish.

"Don't worry."

And do you know, I felt as though I just wasn't going to worry because he had told me not to worry. I felt myself relax and calm down.

"The old is pretty bloody good. In fact your chance of getting better is actually about 80%."

But I thought that 80% was a pretty hopeless chance. 80% to me, meant that my chance of dying, and this was the first time that I had said the word 'Dying' to myself … was 20%. It didn't cross my mind for one single moment that my chance for living was 80%.

"So … we are trying to get results …"

So I was a 'Result'?

" … better. You know if it hadn't been for the trials of new treatments that we have actually been involved with at this hospital, we wouldn't have available what we bloody well do have now … the standard treatments for this illness.

"So … what we would like you to consider … is being involved in a clinical trial of a new treatment for your lymphoma. It could be the future standard, no bloody guarantee mind!"

And then, strangely, he laughed.

Professor Andrews turned to nod at a nurse who was sitting beside him. And bizarrely, such was my level of concentration on the professor, that I hadn't really noticed her presence. Well of course I had seen that someone else was in the room but I had paid absolutely not the slightest bit of attention to what or who that person was.

But at the nod I did pay attention.

Well she was nice … nice and smiley. And she was very pretty. Kind of a bob haircut, brown with blonde streaks and sparkly blue eyes, roundish face and lovely figure. About 5' 5". My age. I know that I should really have been concentrating on our professional relationship … but what the heck, she was very nice looking … and she did have a really lovely figure.

"Caroline, will you explain what we are trying to do?"

"Of course Professor Andrews. We'll go next door. You'll be wanting to get on with the next patient."

The idea that Professor Andrews could have other patients apart from me seemed an outrage. I was his patient and he shouldn't have any others. He should be concentrating on me alone, not wasting time on other relationships. He wasn't to be allowed home until I was better.

Caroline and I sat in the counselling room talking about what would happen next. It was a windowless space cluttered with too many old fashioned pink plastic covered recliner chairs.

"Are you OK so far with what's been going on?"

I was OK. I felt pretty much up to speed with things but I thought that I would pretend not to be so that I could get as much information as possible on board. Also I was pretty worried that I hadn't been told the truth so I thought that Caroline might let me know some of the things that had been kept from me.

"So is it true that that I really have a 20% chance of dying from this or are the odds worse?"

"He's told you the truth. He always does. He's amazing. He's so honest. Too honest sometimes. And he's such a good doctor. You are in the best hands."

Intuitively I had known this, but it was great to hear it confirmed. I thought that I should just sit back and listen to Caroline, and so I did.

Caroline scraped her hair back from her face and pushed towards me a sheath of papers, sliding them across the glass topped coffee table that separated our two Parker Knolls. She crossed her legs, leaned back, and explained that she had given me two sets of information sheets about the lymphoma. The first set she said explained the nature of the illness and its treatment and the second set detailed the clinical trial that I might be involved in if I gave my consent.

"It's a pretty scary document you know. It's written by American lawyers so it doesn't spare the detail! It says at great length what might happen in the worst of eventualities. It really goes over the top. It's put quite a few people off. It's so freaky!

"You really should read it though. And think about things. You must be sure that you want to take part in the study.

"Now … if you agree to be in the study then you will have to sign your consent to take part.

"But … you can only sign after about a week has gone by so that the lawyers can say that absolutely no pressure has been brought to bear on you to be in the trial. And … that you have agreed with full time for thought."

Caroline uncrossed her legs. I remember that she was wearing blue and black striped tights and that her legs were … lovely.

I also remember being really puzzled by the fact of having to sign consent. It seemed to me as though people might be covering themselves in case they were sued by the patients in the trial. It made me think that there were doubts that the treatment was effective. It also seemed to me that it was probable that the new treatment might have terrible side effects which the lawyers and doctors knew about and were worried about.

I was faced with a sudden loss of confidence in the system that I was in.

I remember being really worried, until Caroline said,

"The clinical trial has been approved by the regulatory authorities.

"And … they've been scrutinised by committees of lay people and doctors. They've … made sure that the trial is safe and is being carried out in an ethical fashion."

The worry started to ease a little.

But then I thought 'Why on earth should the ethics of the study have to be considered … is it because the study is actually unethical?'

"This is how it is nowadays. It's all very bureaucratic. But … it's good in a way. Makes sure that everything is above board."

'Above board …' I thought.

"Anyway … you take all the papers away and read them. If you have any queries at all you can ring me on the number on the card."

She handed me a card with her contact details.

"They'll be seeing you in clinic next week to go through things and arrange your treatment. Meanwhile … I'll weight and height you."

I didn't like the idea of being weighed and measured. It was as if I was being fitted out for my coffin.

"And ... I'll book you in to the Chemotherapy Day Ward for treatment."

I began panicking that next week was a long way away and that the delay to treatment might mean that I would die but my thoughts were interrupted by Caroline who said,

"It's all pretty standard for the moment. Do you want me to explain what treatment involves? Or ... would you like to take things a bit at a time?"

I thought that I'd heard enough for the moment. It was about all that I could take on board. I wanted to talk about things to someone who wasn't in the hospital ... and para-doxically, I also didn't want to talk. It was an odd situation really. To talk or not to talk, that was the question, or was it? I really didn't know; I was all in a muddle.

But who to talk to? The one person that I really didn't want to talk to was my Dad. We'd lost touch with Mum. She'd run off with someone all those years ago and never got back in touch with us. Dad had brought us up. He'd been a star, always around for us. Sort of put his own career on hold until we'd left home for college.

No I definitely didn't want to talk to him about anything, didn't want to worry him about me until things were sorted out. Just didn't seem fair.

So, as you can imagine, the lymphoma was preying just a little on my mind. And I really did need to chat to someone. And it never seemed the right time to chat or the right place or person until it just sort of flooded out in a splurge. Came spewing out when I was chatting with Keith, our milkman. I live in a bit of an old fashioned area. Although my flat is in London, the place that I live in is sort of friendly and not at all 'big city'. My neighbours chat, the postman asks how you are, and we have a milkman who does the rounds. Keith the Milk is quite a character. He's about 75 years old, small, skinny and very weather wizened. He's dead conscientious about his deliveries. Never misses a day, unlike our postman who I think has been hoarding our mail for the last six years ... there must be some reason why I never get letters.

Keith is a really nice man. Gives sweets to the kids. He's a menace on that float though. Quite oblivious to the traffic. He'll park his milk cart in the middle of the road, ignoring the hooting horns of the yummy mummies' 4 by 4s. They can wait and they can wait in a line. Keith won't move over. Keith has to deliver the milk.

So Keith and his float pulled up as I was walking down the garden path to get a little fresh air. There was a screech from his handbrake and there he was, walking towards me clinking the red tops. And I said,

"Hello Keith!"

And he said,

"You at home then mate?"

Well of course I was at home and it all just came out in a great avalanche of words as I explained the reason for being off work.

"Oh!" he said, putting the milk bottles down in the middle of the path to our front door.

"You'll be all right mate. Doesn't sound too bad. Where are you being treated then? Where they looking after you?"

I explained.

"It's a good unit there you know, world famous, mate. They'll look after you good and proper. They will. They looked after me brilliant."

I wondered at that.

"Yeh. Had colon cancer, didn't I? They chopped it out and after the op I had no trouble at all. It's been ten years. See. You can get better. I did. You'll be fine mate."

And then off he went and I felt better again.

And do you know that I thought,

'Well, if he can do it I can do it too. Look at the old bugger! He's delivering the milk when by all rights he should be long retired and off clapped up in a nursing home in his dribbling dotage. Best gird up the old loins and get on with things.'

So I did. I got on with things. I started by stocking up with books and downloading piles of stuff onto my iPod. Then I got my washing done. I specialised in stockpiling washing so that kept me out of trouble for a while. I read the stuff about the clinical trial. The explanation was very difficult to understand as it dealt so extensively with the problems that might complicate treatment … so much so that it was almost impossible to work out what the trial was all about.

And before I knew it … well it was clinic time again and Professor Andrews was explaining the treatment to me. Caroline sat in on the consultation.

"They'll put up a drip and give you injections. Then you'll go home. Actually, you should be fine."

I was very puzzled at his brevity. He hadn't brought me up to speed at all. He hadn't talked to me about the treatment and he hadn't explained the trial. It was all quite a mystery

At that point Caroline took over, thank goodness. She waved some booklets at the professor and said …

"Professor, you need to go over the inclusion and exclusion criteria and get him to sign consent."

"Bloody Hell! All right … what do I have to bloody well do then?

"You show me. I can never understand the blasted things."

"Just sign here.

"Tick the boxes professor,

"And then hand it over for him to sign.

"You have read the document? Is there anything that you would like to discuss?"

I had read it of course, and wanted to go through with the trial which offered me standard chemotherapy treatment for lymphoma followed by a transplant programme in which I got more chemotherapy plus or minus a new antibody to suppress my bone marrow. I did have a question for Professor Andrews.

"I understand that the trial is randomised so that I may or may not get the new antibody. I also know that the only way to really find out whether or not the treatment works is to carry out the sort of 'randomised controlled trials' that you want me to take part in.

"But what I don't understand is why it is that if you are randomised to the placebo treatment that you have to go through all the same processes that you would have to go through if you had been randomised to receive the new drug?"

"Bloody good question. I agree with you actually. But that's what the Drug Company asks us to do. The thinking is that if you didn't go through the same processes then other factors might come into play that would affect outcomes. Everyone has to be treated in the same bloody way to make sure that there can be no technical criticism of the result. Got it?"

Needless to say that I sort of got it but didn't get and I signed the consent form anyway.

Caroline smiled and said,

"We've booked you in for treatment tomorrow.

"I'll take you down to the Day Ward and you can meet the team and get an idea of what's going to happen."

So Caroline ushered me out of Professor Andrews' consulting room and into the adjoining Day Ward. It was a ward in the miniature, and divided into two sections. One section contained half a dozen beds lined up against a wall with high round porthole windows. There were patients occupying two of the beds and they ... the patients, not the beds ... looked pretty gaunt and poorly. I hoped to Hell that I wouldn't end up looking like that.

I walked quickly through the bed section of the Day Ward trying not to stare at the patients. The other half of the ward was crowded with recliner chairs, a TV and a nurse's station. There were slightly more lively looking patients in this section, and they were sitting in the recliner chairs. They were linked up to drips and were either chatting with each other, or reading magazines or staring at a muted TV screen.

The nurses were bustling around checking on the drips, laying out treatments, making calls.

"This is Sister Jackie."

Caroline introduced me to a tall woman in a blue nurse's uniform. She smiled at me and shook my hand.

"I hear you are for R-CHOP tomorrow."

This was news to me.

"Yes ... he's for R-CHOP," said Caroline.

"I … haven't gone in to all the details …"

"Don't worry. I'll go through things with him. Come and sit down."

So I did as I was bid. Sat down with Sister Jackie who quietly explained that I would come in tomorrow to the Day Ward, have a drip put up and then have my treatment given through the drip. She explained to me that the drip was up for a couple of hours and that I should be prepared to wait around for most of the morning as the drugs needed to be made up in Pharmacy following the Day Ward order. She told me that people used to be very sick with the sort of chemo that I would be given but that nowadays there were marvellous drugs that stopped the sickness and I should be all right.

"Only trouble is that the anti-sickness drugs can make you pretty constipated."

It all seemed pretty straightforward.

"Oh … by the way … have they explained about neutropenic sepsis?"

She peered earnestly at me.

I had absolutely no idea what she was talking about …

"About seven to ten days after chemotherapy you can get infections. It's because the chemo affects the bone marrow where your white blood cells are made … you know … they're the cells that are part of the body's defences against infection. Chemo stops all cells in their tracks … you know … sort of stops them being made. So if you have no white cells then you can be very poorly with an infection that your body would have no trouble with dealing with normally.

"So … what happens? Well! You'll feel as though you have the most terrible flu, with a sore throat, temperature and muscle aches. Point is that if this happens then you need to come into hospital and get sorted … you know. We'll treat you with antibiotics and you'll be fine. But just remember … if you ignore the symptoms then you can die. So don't you do that … PLEASE!"

And Sister Jackie wagged her finger at me in a most friendly way and me … well … I got the point that it was important not to bluff it out if I was unwell.

"So, call us if you are poorly."

Sister Jackie gave me a little information booklet with contact numbers and my chemotherapy detailed. The side effects of my chemotherapy were outlined in brief with a clear outline of what to do if I had any trouble.

She then asked me to give my signed consent to treatment, which of course I did.

'What are the alternatives?' I thought and was surprised to find myself laughing.

I didn't sleep at all well that night before chemo. I had a terrible dream in which I was floating out of control on a bobbing raft battling with brutal white waters and tumbling down high waterfalls. I really felt those waterfalls. I was drenched in the flume, smacked by the waves. I writhed in the rapids in fear for my life. The water was wild. I banged down into the cold waves, and was thrown up against razor rocks. The dream physically shook me. I was there, it was real. My muscles throbbed with the effort of clinging on to the raft.

I woke with my hands clamped around the mattress hanging on for dear life … and that I suppose in retrospect, that was exactly what I was doing.

The day went quickly. A tiny prick and the drip was up. I was given three injections into the drip.

Sister Jackie explained,

"Some of these injections are to stop you feeling sick and one of the injections is chemo."

She then turned to the drip stand and swopped the bag of clear drip fluid for another bag of equally clear looking fluid which had a big white label stuck to it.

"It's the first bit of your chemo."

The clear fluid felt cool running through my veins, a very bizarre sensation. The fluid was dripped in over a period of about an hour. Then the drip bag was changed and a sinister looking bag of red fluid was exchanged for the clear fluid. I didn't like the look of it, it looked evil. Sister Jackie noticed my anxiety.

"It's called adriamycin."

I really hated the look of the red drug.

"Then, the 'Rituximab.'"

I clearly must have looked very confused.

"It's an antibody against a molecule on the surface of your lymphoma cells. It targets them, knocks them off and improves on your chance of getting better. We didn't use this a few years ago. Clinical trials have shown us that patients have a better chance of surviving if they have the antibody and now it's pretty much a standard add on to the chemotherapy of lymphoma."

I remember thinking …

'Surviving! I like that word. Better chance … I'll go for that then.'

Then it was over and with smiles from the nurses I was off, clutching my bag of anti-sickness drugs and the steroids that were part of my treatment that was to continue for the next 10 days.

I thought that I might be able to make it to the office but it wasn't possible. I just felt a bit stuffed. My GP called me in for a chat. Kind of him, and then he signed me off work for the next couple of months, which was dead nice of him, but that really worried me because it made me think that I was going to get to be like the poor people in the beds in the Day Ward.

So, I took my anti-sickness drugs for the next three days and Sister Jackie was right, they did make me very constipated. Almost worse than being sick I thought. And part of the recipe to control the sickness was a drug called dexamethasone, which made me feel as though I was on speed. I could hardly sleep. Still the drugs did the job: I wasn't sick. It was a triumph of modern medicine! I was really, really relieved that I wasn't too poorly. Made me feel that perhaps I would be able to cope on my own. I managed to get out of the flat and buy the newspapers. Not that I read them. And some ready meals. Not that I ate them.

So, all was going hunky dory, and maybe, I was getting a little cocky because I was thinking to myself that perhaps a week had gone by since chemo and maybe I could get down the road to the pub.

Uh huh.

There was someone up there sitting on a rain cloud wagging his finger at me and … saying …

'NO, NO, NO.'

I woke up with a really sore mouth. There were ulcers on my gums and cheeks. The corners of my mouth were cracked. Then before I knew it, my arms started to quiver and shake. I felt hot and then very cold and started to sweat.

I knew that was what I had been told to look out for. My white cells were low and I had to get back to hospital.

I called the Day Ward and they told me to go to Casualty, and expect to be admitted. I was to tell the nurses in Casualty that I was an Oncology patient and was expected for admission.

I was amazed at the Casualty experience. They were waiting for me. They took my temperature, blood pressure and pulse, and then they got a doctor to come down to see me within about 20 minutes. I was booked in by the doctor, had blood tests and an X-ray, and within an hour of arriving I was sitting in the ward having had injections of intravenous antibiotics.

What a service; it was Rolls Royce.

And do you know I felt better, until the nurse booking me in to the ward said,

"Next of kin?"

That got me thinking.

"We need to know who to contact in an emergency."

There was nothing for it but to tell the family. Not my Dad though. It would have to be Jenny, my sister.

We'd been so close in childhood, thrown together by the divorce, made to rely on each other for comfort and company. But then she'd got a boyfriend and I was just the little brother who was sort of in the way and a bit of an embarrassment, and next thing she was gone from my life … she was off to university.

We'd kept in touch of course but it wasn't the same. I really missed the loss of our *closeness* …

"Jenny King."

There, it came out.

"And her contact details please?"

I gave them.

The nurse looked at me enquiringly.

"Would you like me to tell her you're in …?"

That wouldn't have done at all.

"It's OK, I'll call her"

I did call her. It was one of the most difficult conversations of my life. It made me cry. Not sure why. She was cross with me. Of course I understood that.

"You should have told me," she said,

"I'll come right away."

She came in about 30 minutes and sat in the ward by my bed looking, well … just beautiful I thought. Wearing a sort of a mix of styles that gave her … her own unique style, lots of bracelets, Blackberry clutched in her hand, short skirt, beaded thrift shop cardigan, huge mass of hair, all the shades of blonde and brown.

"How are you?" she said.

"Fine. You're not to worry … they're sorting me out."

"Tell me again what's wrong."

I told her.

"I'm going to be alright. 80% chance. Honest."

"Have you told Dad?"

"No. Didn't want to bother him."

"Are you completely crazy? He'd be so upset …"

"Do you need anything?"

"I forgot my iPod."

"Give me your keys and I'll get it for you."

So she did. And after a couple of days of antibiotics my mouth started to heal and the fevers died away. My appetite seemed to belong to a wolverine because of the steroids that I was taking as part of the chemo. And no matter how gross the hospital meals were, I still wolfed them down, gobbled up the boiled potatoes and sweetcorn, food, designed it seemed, to put a normal person off eating. Weird drugs those steroids.

There were ward rounds twice each day, parades of the doctors who went through my results and checked my charts. Didn't seem to be much continuity of medical care because the doctors were always changing shifts. Apparently it was all to do with the European Work Time Directive which laid down conditions of work. The juniors weren't allowed to work for more than 48 hours each week. I was amused to learn that the Directive didn't apply to the seniors though!

"Time to go home big boy."

This from a rather cool junior doctor, a George Clooney clone. I liked him.

"You've got your appointment for your next treatment?"

I had been issued my appointment for my next chemo course from the Day Ward. Well … I can tell you that I was off and out of there, very, very, very, smartly. I had jumped out of bed and was getting dressed before he'd completed his sentence. I was out of bed before he'd had time to draw the curtains around me so that I could dress without making my neighbours on the ward feel inadequate.

Back on the bus to find that my flat had been invaded. There was a feeling that wasn't quite right that greeted me as I turned the Chubb. It was the smell. Everything seemed fresh. I prowled into the sitting room. It was tidy. The windows sparkled and the flat seemed brighter. The flat was warm. There were anemones in one of Keith's milk bottles on my dining room table and about ten get well cards. There was food in the fridge. The get well cards got me. I found myself blubbing. Hadn't thought anyone cared for me.

There was a note taped to the TV.

'Love from your big sister. Beeeeeg kiss.'

And an impression of bright red lipstick lips endorsing the love.

There were another ten days until my next chemo. The days passed. My sister phoned every day and texted twice a day. Every other day she'd pop in after work. Dad called and then came over. We hugged, something that I hadn't done, I realised, since Mum left.

I found it good to have noise around me. I had the radio on a lot, and the chatter and music distracted me from any morbid thoughts. Believe me there were plenty of those. I seemed locked inside a closed circuit of questions that had answers that looped back to the questions.

There was the 'Will I have to be admitted again with an infection?' question motor racing circuit. The answers to this question were:

1. 'Yes',
2. 'No'
3. 'Maybe'.

If in my mind the answer was 1, 'Yes', I would enter the motor circuit to encounter three stage points. They also had numbers. There was the:

1. 'What happens then if I am admitted' starting grid … which took me to the …
2. 'What will happen in the ward the next time, will I die of infection, hope not?' black flag waving all the cars to a halt point at the crash at the chicane … which brought me to the …
3. 'Probably be OK', chequered flag and then round again to the …

'No' sequence or the 'Maybe' sequence, all of which were really sticky questions because their answers led on to more and more curling chicanes of confusion. So, when I got stuck I would put the radio on and try and drift off on Desert Island Discs or Gardener's Question Time or good old brainless XFM.

But still the musings continued. Particularly in the night. Horrid, just lying in bed thinking. The worst of all of the musings was the 'Am I going to get better?' question circuit. This is one that that if I went into, I would find that I had no numbered answers for. I would just freeze. This was a circuit that I couldn't move around. I would get stuck.

About two weeks after the first treatment day I woke to find masses of hair on my pillow, a thousand spiders on the sheets and pillow slip. What a shock. Of course I knew that I would lose my hair, they'd told me that I would lose it all. But it was still a shock. The hair on the pillow didn't look like my hair. It was as if it had been left there by an old lady. A dead thing, dry and wriggly.

The worst thing really about the hair was that it was evidence of illness. It seemed to tell me that I actually was sick. It was evidence that was incontrovertible and could not be denied. Needless to say that I dumped the evidence pretty quickly. I wasn't going to have that sort of thing hanging around the house. I bought a beanie. It was grey and ribbed, and had the letters 'A & R' printed on it. Looked cool funnily enough. I looked sort of tough. Went out and got the matching hoodie.

So it was treatment time again. I liked the nurses in the Day Ward. And there were a few familiar faces amongst the patients. Most of them were much older than me and I took comfort from the,

'How are you love?'

And the …

'How's it going then?'

It was as if I had another support group in addition to the Professor Andrews and me support group.

So chemo time again. Good-oh.

I knew the ropes, I was an old hand. It felt easier.

Sister Jackie:

"How's things?"

"I'm OK."

"Have you got your appointment for the re-assessment bone marrow test?"

"No, should I have?"

"Sure. I'll check. Hold on there and I'll be right back to you."

Now normally when I hear the phrase 'I'll be right back to you' I'm on the line to a call centre and no one gets back to me. But good old Sister Jackie got right back to me and the appointment for my next marrow test was there written on my appointment card. It was booked for the week before the start of my third treatment cycle.

The second cycle didn't have any complications and the haematologist taking my bone marrow test waited long enough for the local to work so that it wouldn't hurt. I was amazed that it didn't hurt at all.

"It'll take about a week or so to process," she said.

"We'll be in touch with the results."

I didn't like the sound of that at all. Seemed almost ominous. And anyway what results was she talking about?

I was in the Day Ward receiving my third lot of chemo when Professor Andrews swept in with an entourage of about 20 doctors and medical students. Jenny was keeping me company. She was sitting next to me as the chemo was going through the drip.

The professor was wearing a very old tweed jacket with leather elbow patches, the sort of patches that weren't an affectation, but were needed to cover proper holes. There was a gold watch chain looped from his lapel button hole into his breast pocket, and in his breast pocket there was the sort of paisley handkerchief that had been popular between the world wars.

Professor Andrews hung on to my drip stand and leaned over me. He swayed backwards and then he swayed forwards. He smelt of red wine and a six cloves of garlic lunch.

"You're all clear. No clone. Bloody good news. I'd go and have a few jars on that."

And with that he strode off, the entourage struggling to keep up.

Jenny tugged at the sleeve of my jumper. She looked anxious.

"What does he mean?"

"I have no idea," I said.

But Sister Jackie knew.

"The lymphoma has cleared from your marrow. You are in remission. That's the first big hurdle cleared."

I got a big sloppy kiss from Jenny. She stood up smiling and zoomed off to buy a huge tin of Quality Street from the hospital shop. She gave it to the Day Ward nurses. She made me sign the 'Thank You' card.

Time went by, it's funny how time goes by, and the things that seem so terrible at the time, well you get used to them and they are just how it is, a way of life; so much so, that the fact that I went through four more chemo courses seemed to me something that was almost humdrum. It was my new way of life.

I didn't get back to work during treatment. I couldn't make it. Just didn't want to go. It wasn't that I felt too ill to work. My GP understood, bless him. I told him the truth. He signed me off long term sick. I felt no loyalty you see to my work … I hadn't got a single card from work, nor even a call, spoke to nobody at all after that first telephone conversation with the office when I told them that I was a bit poorly.

I took the time to think about the nature of my work and what it meant in the grand scheme of things. And my conclusion was that it didn't mean very much dealing in stock options … not in the grand scheme of things, life and death, which is what I was trading in at the time …

So that was six courses in total; all done, and I was booked in to clinic again to see the professor.

"You're still on for the trial?"

That from Caroline. My, she was even prettier than I remembered. What must she have thought that I looked like? Goodness knows. Face fat with steroids, hairless and pale. What a sight. Sometimes I looked in the mirror and couldn't recognise who was standing there looking back at me.

I remember my answer …

" … Let's go for it."

"Great. Any questions?"

And then I said …

"I'll take it as it comes … A step at a time."

"Great."

So she gave me a typed program that laid out the day to day arrangements of my involvement in the trial. I was particularly interested in the end of the program sequence of 'Recovery' and 'Home'.

But before 'Recovery ' and 'Home', there was the marrow priming and then there was the peripheral stem cell harvest and purge and the Hickman line and the high dose chemotherapy. Those bits of the program didn't seem like much fun.

"Could be worse!

"You might have had to have a matched unrelated donor graft with long term immunosuppression."

I told Caroline that I was glad that 'we' weren't going there, and she laughed.

"Right!"

The marrow priming, harvest and purge.

Why was all of this needed? It was needed because high dose chemotherapy would wipe out my bone marrow. The prime, harvest and purge were carried out before chemo and would provide me with bone marrow cells which would be given to me after chemo to re-populate my empty bone marrow and allow me to make blood cells again. Without marrow cells I would make no blood cells and die.

The prime and harvest were a doodle compared with what I had gone through. The prime … a soupçon of chemo which got all my marrow cells into the same point in their growth cycle. Next, I had to wait a few days for an injection of a bone marrow stimulating drug. The stimulating drug fires the starting pistol for my lined up marrow cells to burst into an exuberant growth phase and spill out into the circulating blood. At that point came harvest time when they drained me of a large amount of blood.

The purge. The harvest had separated out the marrow cells from normal circulating blood cells. These circulating marrow cells have the potential to reform and re-populate normal bone marrow wiped out by chemotherapy, and are called stem cells. Trouble is that some of these stem cells can potentially develop into lymphoma cells. So in the laboratory the next step was to purge the stem cells of lymphoma impurities, using an antibody that sticks to any remaining lymphoma cells and kills them.

"Your cell count is fine …" they announced after the harvesting.

By that they meant that there were enough of my own harvested marrow cells in the blood that they had taken, that if given back to me, would home into my bone marrow cavities, and re-populate my bare as bones empty marrow cavities, cavities that had had all life blasted away by the purge of the high dose chemo.

So why were they giving me more chemo? They hoped that this would eliminate all residual lymphoma cells from my bone marrow. I didn't quite understand this as I thought that they had all gone. Apparently it was a just to make sure sort of thing. Quite a big just to make sure sort of thing I thought.

The Hickman line insertion. That was surprisingly OK. The Hickman line is a plastic tube which has a metal needle in its core. The needle and surrounding tube is pushed through the skin on the front of the chest, threaded through a tunnel of tissue underlying the skin and then poked along into one of the big blood vessels just under the clavicle. Then, with a bit of a pull the needle is removed and the tube is shuffled along through the connecting blood vessels to the right atrium which is the first chamber of the heart. The atrium is the receiving room of the heart … it's where all venous blood drains.

The Hickman line is inserted in the X-ray department. The doctors use an X-ray screen to see where the tube is going. You see it's pretty important that it sits in the right atrium and isn't curled up in some other part of the body. It can sidle off into the great vessels of the neck and we wouldn't want that, no we wouldn't want that at all.

So marrow harvested and purged, Hickman line in place, I was admitted to the ward for high dose chemotherapy, a whole galaxy of potions that stomped into my Hickman line. The mix of drugs came in over a five day period.

I was in the cancer ward and my bed neighbours where young men like me. They had leukaemias or lymphomas. They were from all sorts of backgrounds, two came from Afghanistan and Iraq, but the rest were just plain Essex boys. They were either getting chemo, or in the ward because of infections complicating their treatment. We had quite a nice thing going between us. There was a very pretty lady doctor who did the rounds and we had fun with her.

"Doc, I've got tummy ache."

And my neighbour, a white van driver from Chelmsford, pointed at his belly and asked to be examined.

The curtains were drawn around his bed and the belly examined but the doctor found nothing at all strange in the van driver's abdomen.

The doctor drew back the curtains and marched to the next bad boy lying moping in his bed.

"It's my tummy doc!"

Although the fruit and veg market trader from Basildon complained of belly ache, the grin on his face was evidence against any serious pathology. She twigged after that.

On the second day of my admission the ward cleaner stopped mopping the ward floor to contemplate my drip. He put the mop into his bucket and leaned on the handle.

"You get the green medicine, man?"

"No," I said.

"That good. I like you man. Get green medicine you die."

And then off he went on his ward round, with his bucket and mop to check on his patients.

I was sent home after the high dose chemotherapy. Had a couple of days off for good behaviour. They said that I would be in for about two or three weeks all together so I should get a break from the hospital. I just spent the time quietly. Jenny and Dad came over. It was nice.

Then back in. It was just before Christmas. I was admitted to my own room with a shower and loo en suite.

'Posh!' I thought, 'I must be special.'

But I wasn't any more special than any other transplanted patient. I was actually in isolation and all visitors to my room had to dress in surgical gowns, gloves, hair net and masks. They looked just like surgeons. Caroline came to see me to check off a list of questions that were to do with the trial. I was disappointed about that: had hoped she'd just come to see me for … well … you know …

Christmas in the workhouse, I remember thinking.

Next thing? Well the stem cells that had been harvested from my marrow were re-infused. No big. The bag of cells were linked up to my Hickman line and dripped into me. No huge deal. Just a funny smell of sulphur. For a brief moment I thought that we were having a visit from the stinking Devil and his host of fallen angels, but the truth was rather less dramatic than that. Apparently the stench was from the stuff that the cells had been mixed with to stop them clotting.

And next?

A day or so later …

I forget the precise sequence of events because at that time things got a bit blurred but I think that I had the infusion of the experimental antibody. It came through the Hickman line like most of the drugs that I had been given.

I immediately became very hot and flushed. I was light headed and felt faint. I remember looking up from my pillow to a ring of faces that seemed intent and anxious. Apparently I was having an allergic reaction. They sorted me out though pretty quickly … gave me more steroids and some I.V fluids and I was fine. Came around with a big thumping headache but I was OK.

They seemed very keen on counting my days and doing blood tests. My observation charts had the days from the high dose and days from the re-infusion of my stem cells marked on them. The blood tests were usually once but sometimes twice daily.

At about the fifth day from chemo my blood count started to dip. The lady doc told me that,

" … We'll support you with platelets …"

Apparently if my platelet count got below a certain level I was at risk from spontaneous internal bleeding. They had to keep my count up artificially,

"Otherwise …"

Well I didn't much like the sound of 'Otherwise' and so I asked her to be economical with the details.

The platelets were given to me every day for the next week or so. Professor Andrews came in to see me about twice each week during the early phase of my transplant.

He was just wonderful. So enthusiastic and positive.

He would always have some probing question for the juniors …

And then there would be trouble …

"What are the increments like?"

He turned to the junior doctor and stared at him balefully.

"Not bad."

"What do you bloody well mean …? Not bad?"

His face seemed to go purple with rage. He smacked at my charts and then threw them against the wall.

"What the Hell do you mean? They are terrible. When are you measuring the increments?"

A certain incomprehensible mumbling issued from the junior's face mask.

"That's appalling. You should be measuring levels at 20 minutes post infusion.

"And how are you giving the platelets?"

More mumbling.

" …Intravenously I hope."

The junior shuffled uncomfortably. Nobody laughed.

"Give them as a rapid bolus otherwise they'll be sequestered in the liver. There's a one pass effect.

"Got it?

"I should bloody well hope so.

"Who's examined him today?"

Professor Andrews glared at all of the doctors.

"Are you all completely irresponsible?"

Professor Andrews asked to examine me. I took off my pyjamas and lay on the bed in my Calvin Kleins. He stared at my skin, front and back and pointed out little red dots on my shins that none of the juniors had seen. Well they wouldn't have seen them because they only looked at the results; they didn't take time to look at me.

"Ophthalmoscope please Sister."

He peered into my eyes.

"Retinal haemorrhage at 7 pm."

He turned to the juniors.

"You can't learn to be good doctor watching bloody ER. I expect a better standard of care. Got it?

"Well I bloody well hope you get it.

"I want to see the bloody increments … I want you in my office with the blasted results … at 5.30."

And with not a word to me he stomped off. I liked that. I was sure that it was an act, an effort at setting standards of care, all done to make certain that the lessons given would never be forgotten by the juniors.

My mouth got really sore. It was just like when I had been admitted during the first cycle of chemo but … a thousand times worse.

It looked as though I had florid cold sores. The sores spread from my mouth to around my nostrils. They were crusted and painful. It hurt to open my mouth and when I did my lips split. It hurt to breathe.

They gave me pills for thrush, which is what, apparently I had, but the pills didn't work. They gave me mouthwashes and they didn't work either.

The nurses took swabs from my mouth and started me on cocaine mouthwashes to numb the pain.

My white count went so low that they almost couldn't find a single cell in my blood.

At Day 8 after the first day of high dose chemo my temperature suddenly went sky high, and I felt even more unbelievably shitty than I had been feeling. I started to shiver and shake. They took blood cultures and they started me on antibiotics through the Hickman line.

I couldn't believe that it was possible to feel so frightful. There I was sores all over my face, covered with little red spots, shivering and shaking, just utterly wretched.

Professor Andrews came to my bedside.

When I saw him come into my room I thought that my number was up because it wasn't his official ward time. I stiffened in the bed.

Red faced and leery he loomed over me.

"Told you you'd feel bloody awful.

"Told you that you might bloody well die.

"Well you might. I said MIGHT … Not WOULD.

"But actually you are not going to die.

"And if you have the bloody nerve to do so then I would personally be bloody cross.

"You wouldn't want me to be cross, would you?"

He checked the charts and looked me up and down.

"What's the Chest X-ray like?"

He turned to the juniors.

"Well bloody get one done then.

"I want to see the bloody film and I want to see it in the next hour. Got it? And get ready to treat with anti-fungals."

And off he stomped.

The X-ray was taken in my room because I was too sick to go to the X-ray department. My fever had got to 40 degrees and I was shivering, sweating and shaking. I couldn't move from the bed and so the nurses came in to help me pee into a bottle. They washed me, turning from side to side to swab at my bits. One held me and one washed me. It made me feel cared for. I loved their touch. It was soothing and calming. They rubbed me gently with flannels and dabbed me dry with towels. I was a baby again.

So another couple of days passed. The doctors were anxious about my blood counts. They wanted the white count to come up. But it didn't come up, it stuck stubbornly at about zero. Recovery was the word that I often heard but there was no recovery and the days went by.

"Why are you waiting for the count to come up?" I asked, as I was being helped by a nurse to get on to the bed pan.

"Because it means that your marrow has engrafted."

There were question marks all over my face.

"That means that the transplant has taken and you are getting better."

I understood. But the marrow hadn't recovered and I was still needing platelets and antibiotics and mouthcare and anti-fungals and the occasional transfusion of red cells too for good measure. It seemed like I was being treated with just about every drug known to man.

It was Christmas Day. Dad and Jenny came up to have Christmas lunch with me. Dad had bought me a present. I couldn't unwrap it because I felt too weak and my finger tips were all chafed.

Jenny unwrapped his present for me.

"Gloves. Thanks Dad."

"They're for when you're better and out of here. Won't be long. It's been snowing and you'll need them."

I doubted that I'd need them. The way that I was feeling, the only thing that I thought that I'd need was a coffin.

"This is from me"

Jenny's gift; Christmas cake and a glass vase.

"For your flat! When you get better you'll need something proper to put your flowers in."

She cut the cake. I couldn't manage it but Dad seemed to hoover most of it up.

"Eating for the family, son!"

My skin started to itch and flake away, dry scales crumbling into my pyjamas and onto the sheets.

And then the itching worsened and my poo turned pale.

"You're a little bit jaundiced," they told me.

'Little bit …' I thought.

' … You're either jaundiced or you're not jaundiced.'

"So we are starting you on higher doses of steroids and another drug to help damp down the rejection process."

This appeared an evil bit of news to me. I neither liked nor loved the idea of rejection.

Christ, the drugs made me feel sick. And I got belly ache which ended in them whisking me off for something they called an OGD. They stuffed a big tube down my throat and looked in my stomach. The tube made me gag. They found thrush and a generalised irritation of the lining of my stomach and gullet. More drugs for me then to help damp down the belly ache.

'Serves me right!' I remember thinking as I was wheeled back from the endoscopy suite.

'The pretty doctor's vengeance for us conspiring to get her to examine our tummies!'

The porters pushed me through the hospital corridors, on my way back to the transplant ward. I was draped in surgical scrubs, and had a face mask tucked tight around me. I remember the stares of the people in the hospital corridors: they stopped walking to gawp at me as I was wheeled back to the ward. It seemed as though they were scared by me. Believe me I was scared by me as I caught a glimpse of my face in the mirror as I was lifted back into bed.

If I had looked weird on steroids in my beanie, during the early days of chemo, what did I look like now? I was at the next stage, beyond Auschwitz, skeletal, puffy faced, the whites of my eyes green, a stick like person, pale and poorly.

I lay on my bed, sobbed, and then fell asleep to be woken in the night by a nurse taking my temperature.

It was a good moment to wake.

She was Filipino. And she was smiling.

"No fever!" she said and drew a cross on my chart just below the latitude of normality.

'No fever ...' I thought ... didn't take much notice and fell asleep again.

I slept through to morning. When I woke up I noticed that my mouth was feeling better. The ulcers were gone and the soreness had lessened.

It was a morning like any morning. They took my blood. Same, same, processes. Drugs delivered and taken. Nursing observations made and registered.

'Goodness,' I remember thinking.

'I fancy a nice cup of tea.'

And I had one. It was a nice cup of tea.

There was a shuffling outside the door.

Then a knocking.

'Funny?' I thought.

' ...They never knock.'

It was Professor Andrews. He walked in followed by his entourage of doctors. He sat on my bed and said,

"Told you that you would probably be all right didn't I?"

He looked strangely pleased with himself.

"Said you'd be bloody ill, didn't I?"

I wasn't sure what this was leading to.

And then I noticed.

The doctors weren't wearing surgical masks and scrubs.

Professor Andrews extended his hand to me to shake, and I grasped it.

"The marrow's taken ...

"You've engrafted."

I couldn't help it. I started to cry.

Professor Andrews shuffled awkwardly and coughed.

"You are going to bloody well be OK ...

"And if you don't bloody well mind I'll have my hand back, thank you very much."

They all shuffled off then and I went home.

" ... And do you know ... since then I've been OK, well I say OK, but I've not been ... you know ... right in my head."

"I see!" And the therapist leaned forwards in her chair, face cupped in her hands, waiting, listening ...

" ... Just not myself, just kind of hanging around ... you know ... waiting.

"The illness was a full time business, there was always something to do, something to fill the time.

"I had a community then ... and now ... I am alone.

"And ... there's nothing. I can't get started again, can't work, don't want to go out. I'm just well sort of ... waiting. Silly really.

"So I've come to see you about that and I wonder if you can help me. You know ... massage therapy, acupuncture, aromatherapy ...

"Can you help me?

"Please ...?"

Chapter 3
Fish Ate My Cancer

It was 9 am on a pale autumn Monday morning in Dr James Fennimore's private patient consulting suite. Dr Fennimore had been at work since 7 am. He liked an early start, liked the walk to work through Regent's Park from his stucco Regency house in Chester Terrace. It was the point in the day when he became free, free to think, free to sniff without being offered a handkerchief, free to slurp his tea without being hectored, and free to remember a time long ago when the nurse that he had loved smiled at him in the morning instead of scowling.

The sun was rising sleepily over the Bentleys and Lamborghinis parked outside the birthday cake terraces of Regent's Park and the coca cola light sparkled on the Park's dew iced lawns. Dr Fennimore kicked at the leaves in the gutters. He liked the spiteful susurrus of the shiver of leaves as the season's fallen span away from the beautiful leather of his Gucci loafers. He liked the beautiful leather of his Gucci loafers too.

'In fact, I like everything.' he muttered himself as he crossed the Marylebone Road.

'Even the traffic …

'I am so lucky.'

Dr Fennimore crossed the road dodging between the cars stuck still in the wodge of traffic. He executed an almost balletic turn as he passed between the cars and giggled to himself at his silliness. He walked along Harley Street admiring the architecture of the houses, the early Victorian Complacent,

J. Waxman, *The Elephant in the Room*,
DOI 10.1007/978-0-85729-895-9_3,
© Springer-Verlag London Limited 2012

the occasional Art Nouveau Frivolous, the 60s Monstrous, enjoyed the beauty of the doorway lights, and squinted at the brass plates hoping to spot his friends' names.

"Good morning!"

Dr Fennimore blessed the dustmen with his trill benison.

The dustmen looked up at him as they threw black bin bags into an untidy pile at the junction of Devonshire Place and Harley Street. They cursed him for a wanker and turned back to kick holes in the bags with their steel capped Doc Martins, a pleasant reminder to the rich of the land that they, the dustmen owned the streets.

Dr Fennimore walked along Harley Street whistling the Ride of the Valkyries. There was a tramp asleep on doorstep of number 47, curled up under cardboard. Dr Fennimore fumbled in his pocket for a £1 coin and tossed it on the step by the man's head. It was Dr Fennimore's way to always give to the poor, he never denied the beggar his change, refused the tramp his pennies. In some way Dr Fennimore imagined that his own life was held together by tenuous strings, strands of ragged cotton that were dangerously frayed. He knew that it could be him on the streets, could so easily be him.

A Ferrari roared through red lights as Dr Fennimore walked up the steps to his house on Harley Street. Dr Fennimore owned the freehold of his Harley Street house, and every time he turned the key in the Banham locks to let himself into the building he felt blessed. The thrill of walking into his own property on Harley Street had never left him. He'd earned the money to put the deposit on the building through private practice and had paid off the 90% of the mortgage,

'Not bad for the son of a Manchester butcher's boy.'

He scuffed his feet on the door mat, and looked into the hallway towards the reception area. There were lilies in a tall glass vase on the receptionist's desk, and the display of flowers had masked the smiling woman that rose to greet him.

"Morning Bridget, how are you?"

"Good Dr Fennimore and how are you?"

"We busy today?"

"Yes. Full list. Your first patient's here. Came a bit early. He's in the waiting room. He's happy waiting … he knows he's early. He's got the papers to read and I've given him coffee."

Dr Fennimore walked through the hallway and peered up at the stained glass dome that topped the stairwell. Fractured tints of light flooded down from the glass cupola into the house and onto a stone staircase that spiralled up through five floors of Eau de Nile and gold painted panelling.

Dr Fennimore pushed open the flame mahogany door of his consulting room, hung his cashmere coat on the bentwood Edwardian hat stand, padded across the Bokhara and sat down at his desk. He turned his computer on and checked his email inbox.

Dr Fennimore tipped back in his chair and ran his hands through the fringe of hair that bordered his pate. He'd been bald since he was 21 years old, but still hadn't come to terms with the loss of his locks. It was always a shock in the mornings when he first saw himself in the bathroom mirror, most mornings he didn't recognise the man that stood in front of the mirror scratching his chest and rubbing his sleepy eyes.

'Funny!' he thought,

'How one maintains in oneself the self image of an 18 year old.'

Dr Fennimore looked around the room and admired his paintings and bookcases, the 1930s Italian bronze that he'd bought from that dealer that he'd treated and the Bacon print on the wall. That print … it was always a talking point. There was coffee on his desk.

'So nice of Bridget …'

Dr Fennimore went over in his mind the deal that had bought him the house. It had been such an effort to find the money, get the banks to back him. It had been a once in a lifetime deal brokered all those years ago with the selling agents of a large property company with a very bad reputation. He'd bought the building at a pretty good price and although he'd not known how he would manage to pay the bills as he'd been so extended financially. But he'd made it work by renting out rooms to itinerant doctors.

'Oh well, better get going then.'

It was the start of Dr Fennimore's morning list, a list that extended to afternoons and evenings six days a week, with Sundays off for good behaviour, Sunday mornings daydreaming in church and Sunday afternoons snoozing in his comfy chair while Lydia fussed around with the channel changer.

He shut down his email, there had really been nobody there that he wanted to write to, and walked to the waiting room to introduce himself to the new patient.

A strikingly gaunt man with rectangular steel framed glasses stood up and shook his hand as Dr Fennimore introduced himself. The grip was dry and firm. The man wore a boulder green Barbour over an open shirt and blue jeans.

"Professor Roberts. Nice to meet you ... sorry to hear your news, hope I can help you."

"I'm sure that you can help me."

Dr Fennimore noted the crisp, clipped diction, noticed also Professor Robert's cadaveric pallor.

"Would you like to follow me into the consulting suite?"

Dr Fennimore liked the idea of being followed into his suite. It conjured to him a certain grandness. All the other doctors who rented rooms in his building had single consulting rooms. He was the only one with a suite, a two piece suite: he giggled silently and was deeply tempted to mince as he walked the deep pile carpeted corridor.

Professor Roberts waited for Dr Fennimore to be seated and then, with a,

"May I?"

... sat down on the faux Chippendale chair in front of Dr Fennimore's enormous partner's desk.

Dr Fennimore had bought the desk in auction at Sotheby's. He was very pleased with the piece, early 20th century, agreed, but very grand nonetheless.

Dr Fennimore looked down at Professor Roberts' notes. The information that he received about the professor was very limited, just a single page GP referral. Not as bad as the GP letters that he used to read all those years ago, when he was a casualty officer, stuck in some ghastly inner city A & E

Department, reading the GP letter over a moribund figure in the casualty cubicle. Those letters …

'Crikey!'

And he shook his head at the memory of the GP referrals that read,

Dear Doctor,

Please see and advise,

Yours sincerely,

No this referral letter wasn't as bad as those letters. But it was almost as brief, and told of some degree of frustration on the part of the GP writing the referral letter.

Dear Dr Fennimore,

I would be very grateful for your advice on Professor Roberts' management. He has almost certainly got a testicular tumour and has been adamant that he doesn't want it removed. He has taken alternative medical treatments and is hoping that this will cure him.

Yours sincerely.

'Crikey …'

Dr Fennimore sucked in his cheeks as he read the GP referral letter.

'Why do they do this to themselves?'

Over the years Dr Fennimore had gathered a reputation as an oncologist who was sympathetic to those patients who had an alternative approach to their cancer treatment. He didn't support their approach, didn't condone their ideas but allowed them the space to do as they wished, gathering their confidence to reach a time when they could see that what they were doing had not been as successful as they had hoped. And at that point, their confidence cupped in his hands, his hope was that they would allow him to suggest an alternative to the alternative approach that they had been pursuing.

Over those same years Dr Fennimore had also observed that for many patients the pace of progression of their cancers was leisurely, benign, and for these patients the alternative approach had been of benefit. It had allowed the patients to feel empowered, to feel in control of a time in their life when all control had been lost.

'A testicular tumour, though, why?'

Most oncologists enjoy the happy ever after feeling that suffuses their being when they see a patient with testicular cancer. This trip up the mood elevator comes courtesy of the information that testicular cancer has become curable. Twenty five years ago testicular cancer killed nearly 1000 men a year in the UK. Now fewer than 70 men a year die from the condition out of the 2000 or so a year that get the cancer.

Generally, when counselling a cancer patient, oncologists know that they need to be circumspect in talking about outcomes. More than anything else the patient wants to know about prognosis and all other points are subsidiary to their major concern about survival. This information about survival chance has to be cautiously given, told with care and sensitivity.

But there is a very different situation that faces the patient with testicular cancer because the caution that generally accompanies any discussion about survival with a patient who has cancer is festooned with brilliantly coloured tidings of joy.

Two alternative voyages of information dissemination are embarked upon for the patient with cancer by his doctor, and they are,

The bad news journey …

"I'm sorry but it is cancer."

And the somewhat less frequently undertaken good news journey …

"I am pleased to be able to tell you that you have a curable cancer and will get better."

The oncologist treating the patient with testicular cancer has the joy of giving his patient the good news story, and knows that the treatment that he will offer his patient will bring a cure.

Dr Fennimore mused over the history of the treatment of testicular cancer. Cure for patients with testicular cancer comes courtesy of a wonderful American doctor called Larry Einhorn who looks a little like Woody Allen and speaks a little like Woody Allen too. Dr Einhorn built on the work of other doctors who had found over many years of investigation that combinations of drugs seemed to cure a small proportion of patients with testicular cancer. Combination chemotherapy was first found to be an 'effective' treatment of testicular cancer in the 1960s but only about 5% of patients were cured. In the 1970s new drugs were developed and a couple of these were put together by a Dr Samuels, who found that the combination resulted in about 30 to 40% of patients surviving. Dr E built on Dr S's successes and added a third drug to the treatment program. Dr Einhorn showed that this new chemotherapy cocktail was amazingly effective, showed that it was so good, that virtually all his testicular patients were snatched from the jaws of death.

A real miracle! Dr Fennimore thought that it was interesting to consider the origins of this miracle which owed very little to the textbook science of cancer clinical trials as practised today. He felt that the current process of new drug development was very bureaucratic and rigidly structured, and knew that many cancer doctors thought that the nature of this process actually limited the chances for a successful new cancer drug development.

The rationale for the evolution of Dr Einhorn's cancer curing cocktail is obscure and the development of his program owes more to serendipity and inspiration than to any process driven assessment system. And the marvel was obvious within months of Dr Einhorn's first patients being treated. They were cured. The program was so clearly successful that rumours of the wonder spread around the world and that wonder became standard treatment before any publication announcing efficacy appeared in the medical journals. That Dr Einhorn's treatment regimen was widely used before printed reports were in press, is a strange concept in today's world of local ethics committees, national drug agencies, pan-national licensing authorities.

Dr Einhorn's treatment program for patients with testicular cancer had become so basic to oncology that it was quite a puzzle for Dr Fennimore to understand why anyone in their right mind would not want to be cured by this regimen.

So gathering himself together, taking a deep breath of the scented air that frequented his consulting suite, he looked up from Professor Robert's GP's letter and braced himself for what would clearly be a difficult interview.

"What I'd like to do Professor Roberts, is to go through your story and find out what I can do to help you."

"Sounds good to me. Lets' get going then."

Professor Roberts leaned forward in his chair and took a notebook out from his Barbour.

"Mind if I take notes?"

"Not at all. Feel free"

"So firstly may I ask what sort of a professor are you, what do you do?"

"I am a professor in media studies at City Metropolitan University."

Dr Fennimore's slightly snobbish hackles prickled and then unravelled on consideration of the subject of media studies and hoisted Dr Fennimore's head way above Harley Street. Dr Fennimore was of the view that the fallow fields of media studies should be allowed to remain fallow. His hackles then exploded and took Dr Fennimore's entire body many miles above the city of London, as he felt that the Metropolitan was in fact merely a technical college and unworthy of the title 'university'.

Dr Fennimore continued,

"And can you tell me your story please ... I have the referral letter which is of course excellent."

And the blushes that told of the lie were not in evidence on Dr Fennimore's face.

"It started 18 and a half months ago. I felt a lump. I knew it was cancer ..."

Professor Roberts hesitated for a moment, placed both hands around his face and stroked his bristles. He tugged at his chin and continued ...

"I didn't go to the doctor at first. Kept it to myself. Knew I could keep it under control. Could make it go away even ..."

"So. What did you do?"

"I called a friend. He'd lived most of his life in an ashram in India. He had this guru. I knew he could help me."

"And did he help you?"

"Yes. I am certain that he did help me. He taught me to meditate. That's what we did. We chanted, and we carried out visualisation techniques. His guru chanted for me too. Did it for me in India. He was very helpful."

"What was the process?"

"I established a deep state of meditation. I imagined that I had microscopic purple fish with razor sharp teeth circulating in my blood stream. The fish swam to my tumour. They nibbled at it. The fish ate my cancer."

"After a couple of months the tumour had stabilised. I am sure of that."

"You were sure?"

Dr Fennimore knew that some variants of testicular cancer were very slow to grow. Sometimes, the rate of change of these cancers was so yawningly leisurely that their development could be traced back over five years or more.

Dr Fennimore knew that the meditation hadn't slowed down the rate of growth of the tumour, but rather that the tumour wouldn't have been expected from its natural history to have grown significantly during that time. He also knew from Professor Roberts' few words that he was likely to have a type of testicular cancer called a seminoma.

Testicular cancer can spread to lymph nodes in the pelvis and abdomen and to lungs, liver and brain. Most people with spread of disease have symptoms from the spread. Dr Fennimore was itching to ask Professor Roberts the questions that would allow him to find out if the tumour had spread, but the time hadn't come for questions. He knew that a relationship had to be built before the questions could be framed, knew that those questions if sensitively delivered would ultimately guide Professor Roberts to the treatment that he needed.

Dr Fennimore was a perceptive physician, and understood implicitly that the glue that bound the doctor patient relationship required time to ooze out of its tube and set. The glue had another name … transference, and that name encompassed a white magic that circles between the doctor and the patient, a magic that establishes in the patient's mind all sorts of qualities in his doctor that his physician probably didn't have.

Dr Fennimore hoped that in time the development of positive transference would allow confidences to be exchanged, and ultimately allow the idea of treatment to be accepted by Professor Roberts. Transference is a two way process and within its bounds there are also effects upon the doctor as well as the patient. The doctor attributes qualities to the patient that the patient may or may not have, the doctor becomes fonder of the patient than he would do or perhaps should do in a 'normal setting'. The doctor has to be careful of the transference that's set up because he can find himself overstepping the boundaries that mark the professional relationship.

"May I ask? What is your view of meditation?"

The question shocked Dr Fennimore. He had felt comfortable in his position behind the desk, he felt safe there, shielded and protected, secure in a position of power and authority. Dr Fennimore felt with a degree of indignation that was about to give him indigestion, that it was he and not the patient that asked the questions.

"What do I think?"

"I think that if it works for you, go for it."

"But you haven't told me what you think. You haven't given a view. Do you think it works?"

Dr Fennimore wanted another cup of coffee.

Dr Fennimore felt uncomfortable. He considered that it was a bit early in the morning for him to have explain his position on such matters.

Dr Fennimore felt put upon. Why couldn't Professor Roberts be a good boy and answer his questions?

Dr Fennimore felt that things were getting a bit out of control. In his view there were ways and ways of conducting medical appointments and Professor Roberts' methods were not located on his planet.

Dr Fennimore sat forward in his chair and leant on the desk with both elbows firmly planted in his desk blotter.

Why I haven't even taken a proper history! But if that is what he wants …

"It sort of works, but not on the tumour."

"Meaning?"

"It gives peace and tranquillity but there is no evidence that translates in to any reduction in the size of your cancer."

"But I have evidence that it has helped …

"I could see the aura around the tumour change. The aura went from purple to muddy brown. Meditation stabilised the growth."

"That may be what you think but in my view you have a tumour that grows very slowly indeed. What you have observed is the relatively benign nature of your cancer.

"May I continue?"

"Of course doctor."

"There have been scientific studies that show that meditation does not have any major effect upon cancer … it doesn't make it go away."

Professor Roberts leaned forward on his chair to a point where both men seemed almost to be touching foreheads. He relaxed again and sat back in his chair.

"Doctor. You have to look at who conducts the studies. You have to asses their motives. The studies on meditation were conducted by interested parties. Scientists benefit from disproving alternative approaches to cancer control. In fact, doctor, they are people who in my view and in the view of my friends, have everything to gain from disproving that alternative approaches to cancer control work. They are paid to perpetuate the myth of the ineffectiveness of alternative approaches to drug treatment. They are people that work for drug companies, and if they were to show that non-profit generating treatments like meditation worked, then of course, they'd be out of a job, grants stopped, salaries terminated.

"Besides, this is beyond science. Science does not have the tools to measure the effects of meditation."

Professor Roberts' conversation had become animated and his manner expansive as he warmed to a well rehearsed familiar theme.

Dr Fennimore sighed. He'd long ago tired of hearing conspiracy theory stories about the bias in science.

"Look, I think that we are just going to have to agree to disagree here. Shall we move on, if that's OK and talk about something else? I really don't feel professor that we will be able to come to a consensus on meditation. What do you think? Shall we move on?"

"OK. You are, after all, the doctor and I am just the patient."

"Good-oh!

"So let's continue shall we? That took you through the first few months ... what happened next?"

"Well it began to grow again. It grew, doctor because I wasn't paying enough attention to the proper way to conduct meditation. I was rushing, trying to complete my work, you know, I had the wrong balance and I needed to get things right. So I went to India for a couple of weeks and lived in the ashram. That time out was really valuable.

"Doctor, that worked. I am absolutely sure that the intensive mediation worked for me. But when I came back to London ... the tumour just got out of control again. It grew, I could feel it growing. There were electric shocks that seemed to come out of it. You'll not believe me but I felt them.

"When I looked at my cancer I could almost see the currents. It was as if there was a cascade of sparkling electricity around the tumour."

"So what did you do about that?"

Dr Fennimore knew that there was no way that he would be able to get to the questions that he wanted to ask. He was resigned to the fact that he would just have to go with the flow.

"I found a healer. He was marvellous. That rare thing. A truly spiritual man."

Dr Fennimore tried very hard to warm to Professor Roberts.

"Where did you find your healer?"

"I was recommended to him by a friend."

"And where does the healer practise?"

"I had to go up to Norfolk. But that was a good trip. It took me out of my normal bag, made me think, put me to rights in a way.

"The healer, my healer, lived in a small house in a tiny village a few miles from Sudbury. I rang the doorbell, and it was just amazing … the door opened instantly! It was as if he'd had a premonition that I was there. Doctor, that man has extraordinary extrasensory abilities.

"The moment that I saw him I could tell he was going to be great. He was a tall, learned looking man. He seemed immensely spiritual. It was difficult to tell immediately, how old he was. He had that look. It was as if he could have been 30 or 70. His hair was very long and very black. His face was very lined. He had round, gold framed glasses. He wore a short, embroidered high collared Chinese jacket and matching trousers. His feet were bare.

"I crossed the threshold. He welcomed me, saying,

'I can see that you have travelled with great troubles …'

"His voice … it was so completely understanding of all my problems. He welcomed me to his house. The curtains were drawn. We went into a sort of reception area, a study. The lights were dim. The first object that I noticed was a phrenology head on a coffee table. Then looking around, I saw so many interesting things. Many of them looked as though they came from India. There were wood carvings and stone sculptures, and antique silk hangings. Really lovely stuff.

"And there were cats. Lots of cats. And they were all just sitting quietly. Cats only stay around for someone special.

"I forgot to mention … there were amethyst crystals just everywhere in his house. It was amazing. Amethysts radiate tranquillity. You knew that of course? By the way, you never really own amethysts you know, just borrow them for a while. And then there were the joss sticks. Fantastic environment."

"So you felt comfort there, and had rapport with the healer?"

"Oh yes. But let me tell you what happened next …

"We were standing together and he asked me to take my shoes off and come into the centre of the room. I came into the centre and noticed that I was standing in the middle of a circular rug. It was shag pile, yes, I remember it so well, it was shag pile and it was purple, except for a blazing white rim. It looked like … well it looked like a purple sun."

"What was your healer called?"

"Michael de la Rondue. But he asked me to call him Isfahan."

"Ah."

"And then Isfahan placed both of his hands upon my shoulders and looked me deeply in the eyes. It was as if he was searching for something in my soul.

"He said …

'You've been on a journey, a long journey, and now you are here and you are safe.'

"They were wonderful words Dr Fennimore. I did feel safe, safe for the first time in all of my life. Yes I was safe."

"I can imagine just how you must have felt,' said Dr Fennimore, not believing his own hypocrisy as he heard the words stumbling from his mouth.

"And what did he do next?"

"He said that he would like to help me but that it might take him some time to make the right connections and he would need my help in establishing the neuroleptic responses to my condition."

"What did he mean by neuroleptic?"

"I would have thought that you might have known about neurolepsis Doctor Fennimore?"

"I am afraid that I don't."

"Isfahan has written a pamphlet about the subject. Well I say pamphlet, but it's more like a book."

Dr Fennimore was aware of the length of time that the consultation seemed to be taking and was keen to draw proceedings to a close. He sneaked a look at his computer screen to check the time.

'Damn that wretched machine and its blasted screen saver. I can't exactly look at my watch to tell the time … or can I?'

And Dr Fennimore folded his arms over his chest which pulled his cuffs up just enough for him to see that there were ten minutes left of Professor Roberts' allocated time.

"So what happened next? It all sounds so very interesting."

"It was more than interesting doctor. I swear to you that the man saved my life."

"He said that he was going to try to heal me. You'll remember that he was standing in front of me with his hands on my shoulders. Next thing I knew he'd swung me around and we were in a line, both of us facing the same direction. In front of me there was a red light half way up the wall. It was a circular light. It looked like a ship's bulkhead light, you know, one of those brass bound, domed lights? But instead of the usual white light, the light was bright red. It seemed to pulse. It pumped out light.

"Isfahan kept his hands on my shoulders and talking in a low pitched, quiet voice, a voice that seemed without modulation, asked me to concentrate on the light on the wall. He asked me to keep my eyes fixed on the wall and not move them.

"Then he said …

'I want you to focus on my voice and listen to what I say. I want you to relax, think of my voice, just my voice and continue to concentrate on the light in front of you.

'I want you to feel very calm, very peaceful. And now I want you to imagine that you are on a beautiful beach in a warm country. All around there is white sand and sea. You are walking along the sand towards the sea. You can feel the grains of sand crunching under the soles of your feet. Now you've reached the edge of the beach and have stepped into the water. The sea is lapping at your feet and the sun is shining. Can you hear the water? Can you sense the warmth of the sun on your body?'

" … And you know Dr Fennimore, it was as if I could feel the water."

'Well he would, wouldn't he?' mused Dr Fennimore.

'Of course he'd feel the water. He'd been hypnotised. Wonder what the charlatan did next? More purple mumbo jumbo, no doubt!'

"Dr Fennimore. It was amazing I was really there. I stood on that beach. The sun was on my back. The sea was at my feet. I could feel the roughness of the sand.

"Dr Fennimore, Isfahan then explained that as part of the healing process he would like to treat me with crystals. He told me that I would experience a very great heat and then become utterly tired. Do you know what he did next?"

Dr Fennimore could only imagine what Isfahan would do next and speculated that it was increasingly likely that what he might do would definitely involve the donation of money to a noble cause.

"Do tell."

"Thank you. I am sorry to take up your time. But, I can sense that you're interested and would really like to hear what happened."

Dr Fennimore nodded.

"Isfahan took up a great clump of amethyst crystals. There were about 100 crystals all clustered together. The rock was the size of a joint of pork."

The joint of pork seemed rather out of place to Dr Fennimore. He would have understood the comparison with a slab of smoked tofu, but definitely not a joint of pork.

"He raised the crystals over my head. Told me that he would rotate the crystals in a clockwise direction for 26 passes mirroring the 26 cycles of the sun around the cosmos, and then he would change his approach to an anti-clockwise direction covering all possible meridians and ley lines. He said that this would drain dark energy from me into him. It would leave me weakened. He told me that the process would not involve any pain but that I should feel intense heat above my head.

"He chanted gently as he enclosed me within the meridians. And do you know Dr Fennimore, as he chanted I did feel great heat, it was as if my head was on fire. He stopped chanting, not suddenly but slowly and the pitch of his chanting decreased as the pace of the chanting slowed."

Dr Fennimore felt that it was time to nod again and did so.

"And then his voice quietened all together. It seemed like the room was entirely empty."

'Yes,' thought Dr Fennimore, 'Emptied of all rational life.'

"I felt exhausted. I stumbled. I was so tired. I just had to sit down. And I felt calm. Very at peace. Drained of anger, drained of resentment, in fact drained of any emotion. All I could do was just be."

'Yes.' reflected Dr Fennimore. 'Post hypnotic suggestion. It's a wonderful thing.'

"And I felt that Isfahan was on his way to getting me better. I could feel the tumour throbbing, it was as if it was being rejected by my own immune system. Isfahan had made my body's defences energised, and that Dr Fennimore, is the basis of neurolepsis."

"So what happened next?"

"Isfahan said that the session had finished but if I would like to have a cup of herbal tea with him he would show me his garden before I left. It was a very pretty garden. I noticed that there weren't many cultivated plants in the garden, and what was growing there Dr Fennimore, was allowed to grow without any attempt to restrain growth. There were quite a lot of brambles. Isfahan liked brambles, he said that the vigour of the brambles symbolised the earth's struggle against man.

"Then he ordered a taxi for me. Oh he was very considerate. Wouldn't take any money either. I insisted and he said well if I wanted I could make a donation to the Foundation. There was a collecting box by the door, and he looked away as I put some money in. I put £100 in the tin. It was the very least that I could do. I wanted to give more but needed to keep some change for the taxi fare."

'Wonderful thing post hypnotic suggestion! I knew that the session would end in an exchange of money,' Dr Fennimore thought.

"Isfahan said that he would not need to see me again but that he would help me by carrying out Distant Healing. I asked him what that was and he told me that he would beam thoughts to me from Sudbury. I would feel pressure when he was healing me. It would be just like the session today.

"I said that of course he couldn't spend all that time on me for nothing, I would have to contribute to the Foundation and he said, so modestly, that all contributions would be very gratefully received, and gave me the Foundation's bank details so that I could set up a standing order should I wish to do so. Wish to? It wasn't just a wish Dr Fennimore, it was my duty. That man is a modern day saint."

The shirt cuff ruffed up. It was time, past time indeed for Dr Fennimore to press that little emergency buzzer under the middle drawer of the desk. Professor Roberts was gazing into the distance enrapt. Dr Fennimore slyly pressed the buzzer and a few moments later the telephone rang.

"Thank you Bridget. I think we've nearly finished our session.

"Professor Roberts. That was an amazing first meeting. I felt that I learnt such a lot from you."

Professor Roberts was brought back into the room by the sound of Dr Fennimore's voice and smiled distractedly.

"Thank you Dr Fennimore. That man gave me such spiritual strength."

"I know. I quite understand. Tell me would you like us to meet again?"

"Do you know I really would like to see you again. I think, and I hope that you won't mind me saying this, I think that I have at last found an allopathic doctor who understands me."

"That's so nice of you … so why not, if you wouldn't mind doing so, fixing up an appointment to see me next week and we can continue your story …

"And, by the way, how would you feel about having a little blood sample taken?

"I'm not sure about that Dr Fennimore. I've been told that having blood taken can weaken me. It can reduce my iron levels. It can affect my homeostasis."

"Sure … you can be weakened if a huge amount of blood was taken, but the body has amazing capacity to make blood, that's how we survive. You know … when people give blood they give a pint a time and the body makes up for the blood donation in a week. We have iron reserves in our body and there's no noticeable effect from just 10 ml being drawn … that's all we'd need from you if you wouldn't mind … "

"Dr Fennimore … just for you. I'll do it just for you. Two tubes mind. NO MORE."

"I appreciate your concerns ... two small tubes then. I'll register that on the computer now and if you'd see Bridget in reception on your way out she'll make the appointment for next week and show you where to go for the blood test."

"Thank you doctor. See you next week."

Dr Fennimore stood up to shake hands with Professor Roberts.

" ... UNTIL NEXT WEEK THEN!"

Dr Fennimore sat down, pushed back in his chair and scratched his neck.

'How is it,' he pondered, that such an intelligent man is so stupid about his cancer?'

But even as he posed the question Dr Fennimore knew its answer. Because in the world of the cancer patient where suddenly everything has become incomprehensible, sometimes it is only the utterly incomprehensible that helps some people survive. In the incomprehensible, there is the mysterious unknown and the unimaginable exists. Where the unimaginable exists, there is hope that the mysterious unknown will conspire to provide a cure.

And so the day passed as most days did for Dr Fennimore, the mornings in consultation with new and follow up patients, reviews that consisted of discussions of symptoms and treatments, scan results and prognoses, the afternoons with rounds of his inpatients admitted to the Oncology ward in the Clinic, and the evenings in meetings with colleagues. Then, home at last, home in the very late evening having been called back to review sick patients in the wards, home to a wife who had given up waiting and gone to bed, home to a meal of cold cuts nestling under cling film on the pine kitchen table, eaten standing up to the accompanying snores of a wet nosed dog curled up in his dog basket.

And so the week also passed for Dr Fennimore, a week of full days, rushed meals and exhausted sleep.

'Why do I work so hard?' he wondered.

But he knew why he worked so hard before the question had been framed. He loved being busy, it was as if he had been programmed that way, programmed to feel anxious if he wasn't working. He loved the rush of work, loved being the centre of things, and loved being needed.

And Dr Fennimore's precious Sunday afternoon also passed, though he was pretty oblivious to its passing, spent as it was mostly asleep in his comfy chair.

It was Monday morning again, another Monday in Harley Street. Dr Fennimore was at his desk, where, in preparation for reviewing the day's patients, he looked first at the display on his computer screen of the results of investigations carried out on Professor Roberts. Dr Fennimore had ordered routine blood tests and these indicated how Professor Roberts' bone marrow, liver and kidneys were functioning. The results of all of these tests were perfectly satisfactory. He had also ordered blood tests that reflected on the activity of Professor Roberts's tumour. Testicular cancer produces chemicals that are secreted into the blood and levels of these chemicals can be measured. These tests allow the oncologist not only to make inferences concerning the microscopic appearance of his patient's tumour but also allow the oncologist to conclude on prognosis.

The chemicals that testicular cancers make may cause specific symptoms. For example female hormones made by certain types of testicular cancer can cause breast enlargement. A pregnancy hormone called HCG is also made by some testicular cancers. HCG causes no specific symptoms but can register as a positive pregnancy test, which can turn out to be a bit of a surprise for a chap. Professor Roberts had given Dr Fennimore permission to carry out these blood tests at the end of his first consultation with him, and the results of all of these tests had been normal.

'So,' thought Dr Fennimore,

'No secretory products … he does have a seminoma then. That would explain things …'

There are two major classes of testicular cancer, seminoma and teratoma. Seminoma is generally very easy to treat because it is exquisitely sensitive to chemotherapy and radiation. Teratoma is not quite so easy but sorts out in the end.

Dr Fennimore thus armed with a clinical diagnosis of a seminoma, went out to the reception area to bring Professor Roberts into his rooms. He noticed that Professor Roberts was draped in scarves and hat, gloves and coat and was sweating profusely. Dr Fennimore was curious to know why Professor Roberts was dressed up for Siberia amidst the glorious warmth that an Indian summer had brought to the capital.

"Cold, Professor Roberts?"

"No, Dr Fennimore, in fact I feel very hot. I'm pleased about that you know."

"Why?"

"I have been to see a therapist. She's explained to me that hyperthermia can sometimes be used to cure cancer. So I am doing everything I can to keep my temperature up. You should see the layers of thermals that I am wearing …"

Dr Fennimore really didn't want to check the thermals. He knew that the body had an exquisite system for controlling and regulating its temperature. Body temperature could not really be altered by piling on the clothes because compensatory homeostatic mechanisms swung into play to increase sweating which acts to cool the body down.

"So how have you been since we last met?"

"Pretty good actually. I told you about the healer. Isfahan is continuing to help me. He's been great. And I have spent a few days in the Gerson clinic."

"Really? You have been busy. What a week you have had … more like most people's year!"

"Yes it was wonderful. I'll tell you about it if I may?"

"I went over to Mexico to stay in the Gerson Clinic. It was an amazing experience. They made you feel so welcome. They gave me time, I could ask what I wanted, be what I wanted. It was great. And the environment, it was wonderful."

"And they helped you?"

"Yes. I went into one of their programmes, the full works, low sodium diet, juices, enemas."

"How did it all work?"

"Doctor … the essence of the Gerson approach is … detoxification. The body needs to be detoxified. How can I explain it to you? Let me try. The essence of Dr Gerson's theory is that cancer is caused by toxins and to get rid of cancer the body has to be detoxified. To do that, well, to put it basically, I had to be cleansed. That required juices, gallons of the stuff, and a low sodium diet, and enemas."

"Juices?"

"Yes, carrot and apple juice, you know, oceans of the stuff. Had to be fresh. They really worked hard preparing it all. Sometimes I struggled to get it all in to me because it was such an enormous volume."

"And a low sodium diet?"

"Yes it has a definite effect on the growth of the cancer."

"And enemas?"

"Yes Dr Fennimore, coffee enemas, they work wonders. They help purify the system and get rid of the cancer."

"How often did you have the enemas?"

"Sometimes four or five times a day. They were quite tiring, as you might imagine, but there was no doubt that they were marvellously effective."

"How could you tell professor?"

"I just knew, I just knew that the technique was working."

"Did you take any medicines?"

"Yes they gave me laetrile tablets. They are natural you know, nature's way of killing cancer cells."

Dr Fennimore thought about nature's way for a moment. Laetrile is an extract of apricot kernels. It has small amounts of cyanide in it. He remembered the studies that had shown that it had no effect at all except on the bank balances of the purveyors of the rubbish, predators on the weakness of poor innocents. There had been such a fuss about laetrile that the American, National Cancer Institute had conducted investigations to see whether or not laetrile had any effect at all on cancer and found that it was strikingly inactive. Laetrile was useless.

"Tell me professor, how did you feel after the stay at the Gerson?"

"Just radiant doctor, radiant.

"I came home glowing. My wife said I was unrecognisable. Must have been something to do with the half a stone in weight that I'd lost out there in Mexico, not to mention the half stone that I'd lost from my bank account …!

"But it was worth it. I felt fantastic. You know I felt after I'd been there that people really shouldn't wait until they get a cancer diagnosis before they go to stay at the Gerson. It's a truly mind boggling elevating experience."

Dr Fennimore felt that it was time to move out of Mexico.

"You do look as though you have lost a lot of weight? Is that deliberate?"

"I am glad you have noticed doctor. I've been on a vegan diet since the day I started out on this adventure. It's done me the world of good.

"I am a very strict vegan. And I've given up all alcohol of course."

At this point Dr Fennimore felt that he would just have to comment. He was bursting to say something and that something just rolled out.

"You know there is really good evidence that diet and cancer are related. This is particularly the case for cancers of the breast and prostate. But … and this is a big but … there is no evidence that changing diet after a cancer diagnosis has an effect on the outcome. This has been gone into in some detail. Patients have been entered into clinical trials in which they been randomised to receive dietary modification or not. There are over 60 of these studies that have been completed and all have shown that there is no benefit to modifying diet once a cancer diagnosis has been made."

"That's the trouble with science doctor; I think that we have to believe sometimes that there is more to life than science."

"I would argue though,"continued Dr Fennimore,

"That if someone with cancer wants to change their diet then that's fine. It empowers the patient you know, gives them back control on a life that has gone so completely out of control."

"There is that aspect doctor. I am glad that you recognise it."

"Tell me professor … how much weight have you lost all together since you first felt the lump in your testicle?"

"About 3 stone. I needed to lose weight though."

"What was your fighting weight?"

"About 2 stone more than I currently weigh doctor."

"You might like to ease up a little on the diet ..."

"I'll see how it goes."

"So you've experienced spiritual healing and you have been to the Gerson, you've tried dietary modification, have you gone for anything else?"

"Yes, lots. You see I am doing my best to heal myself."

"I can see how hard you've tried."

Professor Roberts turned from Dr Fennimore but not so quickly that he couldn't see the flicker of tears drifting down Professor Robert's cheeks.

Professor Roberts blew his nose loudly on a purple paisley handkerchief and turned back to face Doctor Fennimore.

"Sorry doctor ... thank you for saying that ... I appreciate your support. I think though that we have probably had enough for today. Don't you think so?"

"I am sorry to have upset you."

"You haven't. It's just that everyone has been so kind to me and sometimes that kindness ... well ... it just gets to be overwhelming. And the tears ... well, they just come. I find myself just blubbing like a baby. Not done that till the tumour came. I don't know why I am such a blubber pants."

And the tears welled up again. Dr Fennimore pushed a box of tissues across the desk to Professor Roberts who reached for a billowing handful of tissues and blew his noise like a Greek god.

"One thing before you go ... Would you like me to talk about last week's blood tests?"

Professor Roberts squared up to Dr Fennimore as if he was about to receive critical information and was gathering strength to deal with terrible news.

"Yes please."

"Everything was fine."

Tension eased, the shoulders sagged.

"Thank you doctor. I am very relieved to hear that."

"Now Professor Roberts, how would you feel if you had one more test. It would be helpful you know."

"Meaning?"

"I think that you should have a scan."

"But what about the radiation dose? Isn't a scan really dangerous? I have been told that any scans involve a remarkable amount of radiation and could not only weaken my immune system but give me a cancer."

"I do understand your concerns. You have been on a plane this year?"

"Of course."

"Did you know that the amount of radiation that you are exposed to on a flight is about the same as you might get having a scan?"

"No I didn't. I think I'll need to consider alternative transport then, I never really enjoyed flying."

"How about considering not flying for a year and having a single scan instead? If you'd consider that, then your radiation exposure doses might just balance out."

Professor Roberts seemed impressed by Dr Fennimore's logic. Dr Fennimore was also impressed by Dr Fennimore's logic which had taken its inspiration from the carbon trading scheme and was just as useless.

He leaned forward in his chair …

"Dr Fennimore, I like your reasoning. Let's do that scan. Yes I'll do it."

Dr Fennimore completed the request form ordering the scan and handed it to Professor Roberts.

"Usual thing professor, see Bridget and she'll sort out everything."

"She's a very nice woman …"

"She is … the kindest heart."

Professor Roberts stood up to leave and shook Dr Fennimore's hand.

"Thank you doctor."

"Until next week then. Good luck with your scan."

It was Friday night at Le Caprice restaurant in central London. Dr Fennimore's wife had insisted that they go out for dinner. She had booked the table and told him that if he turned up late she would divorce him. She had said that there could be no excuse for cancellation.

"We have no life together. It's all work and no joy. The kids have gone and we do nothing."

Dr Fennimore skitted in to the restaurant, whooshing through the revolving door to greet Jesus the restaurant manager. He loved shaking hands with Jesus. Paul, the Maitre D' looked up from the reception desk.

"Nice to see you Paul."

"Nice to see you too Dr Fennimore. How have you been?"

"Busy Paul, very busy."

"Would you like to leave your coat?"

"Thanks."

"Let me take you to your table. Lydia is already there."

Paul ushered him to the table and as they passed him, the pianist looked up and smiled at Dr Fennimore. Le Caprice, Dr Fennimore loved it. Going there always felt like real going out. Dr Fennimore looked around to see if there were any celebrities there tonight. No. He'd spotted Mick Jagger there once. Mick had looked very lined, and his hair dye... well... it was just awful.

'Oh God. I hope I'm not late.'

Dr Fennimore glanced at his watch. He was wearing the gold Rolex, gift of an Arab prince, a minor scion of the Saudi Royal family. He was marginally late, just 10 minutes or so. He hoped that Lydia wouldn't be too cross with him...

"You're late darling. You're always late. You were never late when we started going out. You were always on time."

He bent to kiss Lydia's cheek. She was wearing black, a tight, rucked skirt and a ruffled silk top. She looked great and he remembered then why it was that he had asked her to marry him. He wasn't quite sure why she'd consented...

"Sorry."

"You're always sorry darling! You're late...

"But you know that I won't be cross with you for long."

She smiled at him and leaned across the table to stroke his arm.

Dr Fennimore loved her touch. He loved her voice, that husky edge to her voice… come to think of it he loved everything about her… still… still!

"I do understand you know…

"Do you know why we're here tonight?"

Fortunately Dr Fennimore did know why they were here. Bridget had reminded him. But a little bit of the Devil slipped into him as he said…

"Yes. You wanted to go out to dinner. You said that we needed to make time for ourselves as a couple."

"Yes darling … there was that…

"Can you think of any other reason for us being here tonight?"

Lydia looked across the bread rolls and flowers and waited for his answer.

Dr Fennimore smiled at her and then, waiting just a second or two for dramatic effect, pushed a little black velvet lined box towards her.

"Happy anniversary."

And the frown on Lydia's face became a smile and all was well between them.

Morning came and Dr Fennimore was at his desk again.

"Professor Roberts! Nice to see you again. How are you?"

The two men shook hands and sat down.

"I have some good news for you."

Professor Roberts' face registered no emotion as he listened to his doctor.

"The scans are just fine. There is no evidence of any spread of the growth."

"Ah… so the treatment has worked."

"What treatment?"

Professor Roberts became animated, he grinned, leaned forward in his chair and smiled.

"The treatment… I went to the Eagle Clinic and had ozone treatment."

"What's that?"

"It's a wonderful idea. You see ozone has been shown to activate cytokines which are the body's natural defence against cancer. I had autohaemotherapy. It's so clever. The doctors at the Clinic took a small sample of my blood, exposed it to ozone, and then injected it back into my veins. The activated blood cells then delivered their antioxidants to heal my body.

"So you see… it's working."

Dr Fennimore thought about the remarkable process of utter charlatanism that had completely defrauded Professor Roberts and marvelled at the complexity of his patient's delusions, delusions that had been fuelled by unscrupulous parasites preying on the defenceless. Cytokines are the chemicals that are made by white blood cells that help deal with infection. Altered levels of cytokines are found in cancer patients and can be used as a treatment in extremely high doses in one or two cancers, such as melanoma and kidney cancer. Doses of cytokines needed to treat cancer effectively are the equivalent of a neutron bomb when compared with the small fart of cytokines released by ozone treatment. There is no evidence that the ozone treatment would in any way have any effect on Professor Roberts' testicular cancer.

"Professor, how would you feel if I had a look at the little lump?"

"It isn't that little Dr Fennimore… but it is definitely shrinking."

Professor Roberts stepped behind the antique Chinese screen that provided privacy, shielding the examination couch from any who would look. And if any would look they would have seen a very thin man undressing carefully, a thin man folding his clothes with precision and delicacy, a thin man inspecting the couch and straightening out the paper sheet that protected the couch from the patient and stretching himself out on the paper to lie in his vest and underwear awaiting the doctor's attentions.

"Are you ready professor?"

"Yes."

Dr Fennimore stepped behind the screens.

"I am going to examine you, if I may. I'll look at your hands, feel you neck and then have a look down below if I may?"

"Of course doctor."

Professor Roberts smiled up at Dr Fennimore as the doctor took up his hand. Dr Fennimore turned Professor Roberts hand in his, looking at the fingernails and then inspected the palm. The palm of Professor Roberts' hand was orange in colour.

"Carrots!"

"Beg your pardon doctor?"

"Carrots … when someone eats a lot of carrots their skin changes because the carotene that gives carrots their colour is deposited in the skin.

"Good thing too."

"Sit up for me please."

Professor Roberts sat up.

"Could you lean forward please?"

Professor Roberts tipped forward holding on to his knees for stability.

Standing behind Professor Roberts, Dr Fennimore leant over and examined the base of his patient's neck. He was feeling for lymph nodes but there were none.

"I am examining for any spread of your lump that might not have been seen on the scan …"

"And?"

"There are no enlarged nodes, which is a very good thing."

Dr Fennimore could feel the tension in Professor Roberts ease.

"You can lie down again. Are you comfortable?"

"Yes thank you doctor."

"Would you mind lowering your pants so that I can have a look at what's going on down below?"

Professor Roberts shuffled his Y fronts down and adjusted his penis and testicles. He looked up nervously at Dr Fennimore.

"Go ahead doctor. I'd like you to look. Nobody has examined me since that first time with my GP. It was quite an uncomfortable experience, and a bit embarrassing. I would have preferred to have been seen by a gentleman."

"I can understand that, but you know… women doctors… they may not be gentlemen but they are professional people."

"Sure. It was my problem. I feel good though with you. So what do you think doctor?"

"Let me feel."

Dr Fennimore could see that Professor Roberts had a swollen and distorted left testicle.

"I am just going to examine the good one first!"

He raised up the right testicle a little and rolled it between both thumbs and fingers, running over the surface of the testicle to get an impression of its outline. The testis felt smooth. There were no bumps on the surface. He then examined the epididymis and veins that encircled the testis and found a tiny bump in the epididymis.

"That's fine, you have a little cyst but it's nothing to worry about in any way. May I examine the other testis please?"

Dr Fennimore had felt Professor Roberts tense up again and was concerned that he might change his mind about being examined.

"Certainly. Please do."

The left testis was about three times the size of the right testis, but it was separated from scrotal skin and mobile. Dr Fennimore was pleased with these findings as they meant that the tumour was operable. But the testis was hard in places. It felt craggy and lumpy, with a rim of normal testis tissue at its base.

Dr Fennimore put the testis down and felt in Professor Roberts' groins for enlarged lymph nodes. There were no large lymph nodes.

Dr Fennimore's clinical findings had shown him that it was very likely that Professor Roberts had a curable condition, and that cure could be simply achieved … simply achieved if his patient would accept treatment.

"Do get dressed and then we'll have a chat."

Professor Roberts dressed slowly, his movements deliberate and thoughtful.

"So what do you think doctor?"

"May I ask what you think professor?"

"Well, it's been18 months now and it hasn't gone away completely away …"

Dr Fennimore held his breath.

"And I have been thinking that I would like to go through the list of supplements that I am taking with you to see if you think that any of them in higher doses might work for me, would you mind?"

Dr Fennimore held his breath.

'Good God!' he thought, 'I think he might be coming round!'

And despite his many years in medicine Dr Fennimore found himself excited at the prospect that he might have brought this patient to a point of acceptance of the medical process. Or as Lydia might put it, manipulated his patient to become part of process.

"Shall we go though the supplements then?"

"Please: I have bought a list, you might like to look at the list?"

"I'd be very pleased to do so."

"Here it is doctor."

And Professor Roberts reached in his suit for the list and handed an A4 sheet of lined paper to Dr Fennimore who scanned the list of products. The list was written in green ink in an italic script.

Moducare
Phosdrops
Ecogas
MSM

Anox
Designer protein
Co-enzyme
Mycostat
Xell 02
Milk thistle
Polyzyme
Lipaen
Thyroid armour
Chymopex
Querctin

"Gosh, quite a list of products. I don't think though that you should try them in higher doses."

"OK doctor, thanks for going through the list.

"They are good though, aren't they? And of course there are the vitamin supplements. It's quite a business doctor. Takes me about an hour a day just swallowing the pills. You mustn't rush them you see."

"What else do you do?"

"There are the baths doctor. Hot baths with Epsom salts five times a day; it's part of the cleansing process. And of course I have given up alcohol."

"Any Chinese herbs?"

"Yes I forgot about those."

"You need to be careful about the 'herbs'. Some of them are adulterated with steroids and others can cause kidney failure. You need to be very careful. And you have to watch out for the vitamins too. Too much vitamin A, D or E can be really bad for you… can cause liver failure, kidney failure, the works."

Dr Fennimore saw that his diatribe hadn't really helped the rapport that he had worked so hard to establish and so he backed off a little and said,

"But if you stick to the dose on the labels then you'll be OK."

Dr Fennimore knew that the regulatory authorities were powerless to prevent the sort of abuse and exploitation from which Professor Roberts had suffered because the products that he had bought were registered as food supplements.

Because they were food products the manufacturers were only obliged to test for purity and didn't have to demonstrate efficacy. But the EU had set up regulatory processes that would hopefully control the exploitation.

Professor Roberts seemed to relax again and with this easing of the tensions between them, Dr Fennimore thought that it might be just the moment to re-direct the conversation and asked,

"You mentioned that it had been 18 months and that it didn't seem as though it had gone away completely. So how do you think that we should proceed?"

"Could you advise me doctor?"

"In your situation where you have tried so many things maybe you should just think about a little op?"

Dr Fennimore could see that Professor Roberts seemed interested in the idea and feeling his way gently continued,

"You would be amazed how straightforward removing the lump actually is…"

Professor Roberts remained interested.

"It's done as a day case so you wouldn't have to come into hospital overnight. You would need a general anaesthetic. There are new anaesthetic drugs around now and they are amazingly effective, no hangover, no discernible side effects…"

Dr Fennimore could see from his body language that Professor Roberts had accepted the idea that he could no longer put off surgery.

"And the surgeon is a decent man and a world expert. You'll like him. He's pretty unusual for a surgeon; he's actually quite a sensitive person and amazingly he doesn't think that surgery is the answer to every medical problem. He's one of those rare surgeons who isn't scalpel happy."

Professor Roberts stood up and shook Dr Fennimore's hand.

"Let's do it. But I want it done as soon as possible."

"That's great news. It'll be done tomorrow if you want …"

"I do. I've made up my mind and I want it out."

Professor Roberts had the operation and came for review a few days after surgery.

"You have got a seminoma, which is the best of all news that I could give you. The outlook is more than excellent ... it's brilliant.

"Now we have to discuss whether you want any extra treatment. The reason for the discussion is that if you are left without any extra treatment there is a chance of about 17% that the seminoma could spread. With the extra treatment the chance of it spreading in the future is less than 1%.

"And here is the kick. If you go without the extra treatment now and at some future point things go wrong and the seminoma comes back, well, treatment will cure you then. So in a way your decision is based upon how you feel about both scenarios... treatment now or treatment later."

"Doctor. I'll go for it now. What does the treatment consist of?"

"It's pretty straightforward. Either two courses of chemotherapy or three weeks of radiotherapy treatment."

"Why the choice?"

"Radiotherapy is the conventional treatment and chemotherapy the modern option."

"How does one choose between the two treatments?"

"If you want I could guide you?"

"Please do."

"Chemotherapy consists of two injections given three weeks apart and there are unlikely to be any side effects. The radiotherapy is safe but it is associated with a small risk of late complications. Since the two treatments are of equivalent effect ... go for the treatment with the least problems associated with it."

"OK... but which is that?"

"The chemo ..."

"Oh yes... sorry... you did explain."

"I'll arrange it all for you."

"Thank you ever so...."

And as Professor Roberts got up to leave, one question crossed Dr Fennimore's mind and popped out of his mouth before he could think the better of asking it.

"Tell me professor, why is it that you took the alternative medicine route and now have gone so wholeheartedly for conventional medicines?"

"Belt and braces doctor. I'd thought that I would like to have everything."

And as he turned to leave Dr Fennimore could have sworn that he saw Professor Roberts wink at him.

Chapter 4
Smoker's Cough

Nervous Jeffrey. Nervous Jeffrey M. Jeffrey, who had never married, Jeffrey who had never managed to work, Jeffrey who had never quite grown up, Jeffrey with an IQ of 85, Jeffrey who had lived with his mum until he was 52 and then on the day after his 52nd birthday, when he had started coughing blood, had moved out of the family home, moved to a hospital bed, and there in that hospital bed languished, awaiting his fate.

It was a bright autumn morning, and Dr Simon Green, a junior house doctor, had completed his tasks. Blood test forms had been written for the phlebotomist, his rounds of the patients had been completed and his blessings had been dispensed to the nurses. He left the ward for Casualty, as Jeffrey was wheeled into the ward on a trolley, pushed to his bed from the X-ray Department. Dr Green was rather good looking and was aware of his good looks. He was wearing a short white doctor's coat over corduroys, button down shirt and thin tie.

Dr Green was the junior doctor on the 'Cancer and surgery firm.' Firm structures and personnel were fashioned on a model of medicine that hadn't changed since the 19th century and bore the brush marks of the Middle Ages. There were the consultants, who would condescend to consult from busy private practices. There were the registrars who in past times were meant to register and record practice but who in a more modern age ran the day to day business of the firm.

J. Waxman, *The Elephant in the Room*,
DOI 10.1007/978-0-85729-895-9_4,
© Springer-Verlag London Limited 2012

And then at the bottom of the heap were the housemen. The housemen and women executed the business of the firm and by all means it was in many ways an execution. The houseman's on call duties have only recently changed. Dr Green was on call one night in two. This meant that he started work on a Monday morning, worked through Monday night and Tuesday, and only then, at the end of the normal Tuesday working day was he allowed to return home. Back to work on Wednesday morning and back home on Thursday. Thursday night off and back to work on Friday morning and through without a break to Monday evening. Seems a little bit of a strain in the context of the European Work Time Directive. 120 hour weeks! They did happen!

It was the houseman's job to book in the patient, arrange blood tests, organise X-rays and prescribe medicines. On a surgical firm 'Theatre lists' were also prepared by the housemen and these were lists of the day's operations and patients. The operations came first and the patients followed. The most important aspect of the houseman's role was to keep the nurses happy. Good relationships between nurses and doctors made for a happy ward and on a happy ward the consultants got cups of tea and biscuits and the patients never died. Simon Green excelled at keeping nurses happy. Simon's friend Colin Trask was also brilliant at relationship building with nursing colleagues; he built whole cities of relationships. His building works were so time consuming that he would have to wake his patients up in the middle of the night to book them in for surgery, because he had been so busy in the day erecting relationships.

Simon's registrar came from the North East. He had not gone to public school and wasn't very good at rugby.

Joe Peters. Mr Peters.

"Do you know what it's like to look at the docks boy?"

"No, Mr Peters."

"It's not much of a future looking at the docks."

"Yes Mr Peters."

He was definitely right about the docks. Joe was right about most things.

He was also dazzlingly gifted and his abilities were so out-standing that it allowed him to survive in a system that was class driven and really didn't want anything to do with him.

Simon was sitting at a desk in the open ward writing theatre lists. Computers hadn't been invented then but he did have a biro. There were six theatre lists needed, one for Mr Cowie, and one for Mr Worth. Mr Cowie and Mr Worth were consultant surgeons. One copy was also needed for Ward 1:3 and one for Ward 3:1, one for Theatre 1 and one for Theatre 2.

Simon wrote and he wrote. Joe stood on the other side of the desk; he swayed backwards, hand on his chin, then shifted his weight and leant on the desk.

Joe stared with interest at Simon's activities. He watched him write.

Simon looked up and smiled nervously at him.

'What did he want?

'What was he doing?'

It was unusual for Joe to spend so much time in one place.

Joe scratched his head and Simon carried on writing.

The nurses walked by, patients coughed, the phone rang.

Sister answered the phone and Simon carried on writing his clinic lists.

There: he had done four lists, 15 minutes had passed and he was nearly finished. Nearly time to go down to the mess. Simon liked the doctors' mess.

The mess was located in the basement of the nurses' home, a basement with barbed wire draped over a stairwell that denied junior doctors access to the nurses' quarters.

The mess was a one room hideaway, grubby carpet, tatty armchairs, torn curtains, a pool table and piano. To the mess came the mess cook, at 11 am on weekdays and 11.15 at weekends. Cometh the hour, cometh the quarter past the hour, cometh a lardy soul, dressed in grubby whites, chef's tall hat poised at a tilt, a noisy soul, wheeling a rattling trolley loaded with clinking plates piled with peeling white bread and ham sandwiches, a drunken trolley bumping over rucked carpet with its burden of clunking bottles of tipsy pale ale.

The sandwiches and bottles had been bequeathed by a patient to University College Hospital's junior doctors.

In bustled chef, head down, chin in his sandwiches, and parked his trolley with a great crunch into the mess wall, just next to the piano. Every night, the crunch, followed by a great guffaw from chef who would look up at the waiting junior doctors, straighten his hat, stretch his hands, twiddle his fingers, and then sit down at the piano. He'd play for the doctors, always a big twinkly piece, delicately folded from meat platter hands, a single song plucked from a West End show. One song. Slam the piano lid. Bow to the boys. And then he would bustle off to poison the rest of the hospital with the contagion of his grubby fingernails.

Joe was still hanging around. And Simon wondered what he was up to.

Joe coughed, and stared at him, beady eyed, curious.

"What you doing boy?"

"Writing out the theatre lists Mr Peters."

Joe nodded his head.

"The theatre lists Mr Peters. There's one for Mr Cowie and one for Mr Worth, one for Theatre …"

Joe nodded again.

"I see."

"Yes and then there's one for Ward 1:3 and …"

"What you got up here boy?"

Joe tapped his right temple with his right index finger.

Simon was uncertain what he had behind Joe's right index finger.

Joe pointed at the desk.

"And what's in the top drawer of the desk, boy?"

Simon had no idea what was in the top drawer. It was clearly in his best interest to pull open the top drawer. There was a pile of carbon paper in the drawer. It was at that point that Simon realised exactly what he hadn't got behind Joe's index finger.

"What's that on the desk boy?

It was a telephone.

"Think, boy. Think before you do anything, boy."

The wheels of Jeffrey's trolley clattered on the ward's floor boards. At Jeffrey's request, the porter stopped pushing the trolley as he came abreast of Dr Green. Jeffrey, lying on his back on the trolley, head supported from the horizontal by his crooked elbow, turned to look up at Dr Green. Their eyes met.

"Back from X-ray Jeffrey?"

"Yes doc."

"How was it?"

"Well doc, you should know, they tell me nothing."

Jeffrey's many facial mannerisms came into play, the left corner of his mouth lifting to touch his nostril, his nose leering away to clasp at his ear, an epileptic galaxy of winking tics errupting on his face to be chased away by explosive coughing, that ended with Jeffrey spitting into his handkerchief.

Jeffrey inspected the globs of spittle and congealed blood in his handkerchief and then, looked up enquiringly.

"I'll go and find out Jeffrey."

Jeffrey was child like, anxious and awkward, looking up to this callow youth as if he were an authority, and the callow youth responded to his patient's urgent need by going to the X-ray department and inspecting with the radiologists, the films that had just been taken. The X-ray of his chest had shown an enormous mass at the apex of the right lung, a mass that extended right down to the lung's root, which is called the hilum. The radiologist's verdict … an inoperable tumour.

Dr Green came back to the ward and drew the curtains around Jeffrey's bed. It was serious conversation time. Jeffrey sat on the side of his bed, pyjamas adrift.

"What you going to tell me doc?"

"It's not great news Jeffrey."

Jeffrey leaned forward so that his face was too close to Dr Green's. Jeffrey's breath was on Dr Green's cheek and he noted the greyness of his cheeks, the mark of a smoker.

"It's a cancer isn't it doc?"

"Sorry Jeffrey. You're right. I am really sorry."

"You'll laugh at this doc."

Dr Green was not sure that he would laugh. It didn't seem quite the right time for laughter.

"You know how I started."

"Started what Jeffrey?"

"Smoking doc. It was when I was in the bin."

"Really!"

"Yup. One of the doctors there, nice chap, said to me ...

'Jeffrey you know what your trouble is don't you? You haven't enough to do. You need a hobby.'

"And then he said to me ...

'Jeffrey, why don't you take up smoking? It'll calm you down and give you something to do.'

"So that's why I took up smoking doc. To calm me down and give me something to do. That's a fact doc. But you know doc I don't hold a grudge. He gave me good advice. Smoking has held me steady for 30 years. Not bad, is it?"

We have been sure of the relationship between tobacco and cancer for at least 60 years. In 1950, Richard Doll, a medical statistician, carried out a study of lung cancer patients and concluded that smoking was linked to the development of lung cancer. In 1954 he published his observations on the lifestyles of 40,000 doctors and found conclusively that lung cancer was associated with smoking. In the same year, the insidious campaigning by cigarette companies to refute the association between cancer and smoking kicked in. After all, they claimed, it was *just* an association, because not everybody that smoked got cancer. They were right of course, not everybody, but most people that smoked got a nice little present from the cigarette manufacturers; ischaemic heart disease, intermittent claudication. It is likely that we have really known about cancer and cigarettes for many years before Doll. Mark Twain in his autobiography, written over 100 years ago witnesses the final months of General Ulysses S Grant and comments that Grant's cancer must have come from smoking.

In the mid-1960s serious campaigning against the evils of tobacco started to begin, and around that time Dr Green's own father stopped smoking and took up Mars bars and strong peppermints. A lot of doctors gave up smoking in the 1960s but it is unclear how many of them became addicted to

Mars bars and peppermints. As the doctors stopped so their health improved. But it was noted that it took many years for the effects of cigarettes to wear off, years in proportion to the number of cigarettes that were smoked.

Around that time, with revenues potentially affected by the negative reports, tobacco companies started to tap into new markets, targeting women and kids and the innocents of non-industrialized countries. In the UK, the numbers of people smoking has fallen from around 60% of the adult population to the current figure of less than 20%, but with this fall has come an increase in the proportion of young women and teenagers smoking. Cigarette smoking continues to decline in the industrialized world and so to promote sales the cigarette companies have turned to India and China as new sources for income. The companies have supported that drive for income with advertising campaigns and high level lobbying that include as its fatly paid advocates, a former UK Conservative government health secretary.

Cigarette company advertising spend is enormous, with annual estimates in the range of tens of billions of dollars. The ban on tobacco advertising that is applied in the industrialized world took many years to come into play. The initial ban in the UK was on direct advertising and so advertising campaigning became indirect. Indirect was good advertising, indirect drove campaigns forward with an emphasis on branding by imagery. For a time the colour purple was synonymous with fags rather than the clergy, and the cowboy, with cigarettes, rather than the rolling planes of Wyoming. Some irony then when the Marlborough cowboy died of lung cancer and a replacement cowboy was required.

Advertising, in the form of product branding, became an important source of sponsorship for sports, but one by one sportsmen and sports governing bodies were shamed into declining the generous offers of tobacco companies, and the last redoubt of tobacco advertising campaigns became Formula One motor racing and snooker. The branded black car races futilely around the tracks, circling, circling, a metaphor for the predatory tobacco company circling the smoker, the black ball in the final pocket, mirroring the last intake of the smoker's breath.

And what do we have now? How has the campaigning evolved? In our time the ban on advertising has itself become an advertising feature. The cigarette packet stamped with giant warning signs of the dangers of smoking in pregnancy, of cancer, of heart disease, advertises and glorifies the product that it is meant to delegitimise. The warnings make smoking attractive, conferring glamour and the thrill of a battle with convention.

It is clear that the interactions between governments and cigarette companies are delicate. It has taken many decades for cigarette advertising to be banned and the reasons for this bizarre governmental response to the evil weed are hidden in the mire of complex governmental accounting practice. It is indeed a cautionary tale. It has been estimated that if the whole population were to give up smoking then the revenue consequences to government would be disastrous. In the UK it has been argued that the amount of dosh raised by government from taxing smoking is equivalent to the public money spent on the NHS in treating smoking related diseases. The books are apparently balanced. Well er, actually, um, yes, but no, there's little truth in this argument and the defence put forward is a merely part of a malign myth.

The rest of the public accounting myth is destroyed by the truth which relates to the pension consequences to the Nation, of the entire populace stopping smoking. If everyone in the country were to stop smoking, then it is said that the average age of death of the population would rise by a couple of years. If this happened then the consequences for the public purse would be enormous. Our creaking pensions system would collapse. So, every health minister faced with banning smoking completely has had to proceed with enormous caution. Slowly, slowly minister, hang on there with your radical ideas, Excuse me minister, just a minute, hold off Sir, or you'll bankrupt our country.

But the story doesn't quite stop at this point. Those couple of years quoted in the statistics are not quite fact. If we drill down on these statistics, then there below us hidden in the magna, is the pool of enlightenment. Let us walk towards that golden pool. In the 1950s the average age of death of a man was 65 years, a considerable advance on the middle ages when it was in the 30s. But the last 50 years have been witness to further changes in life expectancy. The current average age of death of a man is 79 years and this improvement is not only to do with better health care but much more significantly, due to life style changes and advances in public health. Our walk has taken us to the edge of the pool of enlightenment. Let us now dip our toes in that shimmering pool and focus on life style. The current average age of death for a man who is a non smoker, and isn't obese is 88 years. So wiggling those toes in the water we find another 9 years of life in the shallows. So, put that in your pension pot and smoke it! No wonder there has been some economy with the truth about the truth about the economic consequences of smoking.

Back to Jeffrey. Nervous Jeffrey.

Jeffrey's chest X-ray had shown him to have a large lump at the edge of his lung where it abutted on the major blood vessels at the centre of his chest. This is called a 'hilar mass'. The hilum is an anatomical area adjacent to the heart. The hilar regions are where the mass of blood vessels and bronchial tubes are located that come and go from the lungs to the heart and to the main airways. The hilar regions are like T junctions where the roadways of arteries and veins, lymphatics and bronchi meet and divide.

Jeffrey was booked for a bronchoscopy. This is a procedure where a flexible fibreglass telescope is used to obtain a view of the airways. Jeffrey lay on a bed in the bronchoscopy suite surrounded by doctors, nurses, and a complete galaxy of high tech equipment. With the barest of explanations, the bronchoscopist put a cannula in one of the veins in the back of Jeffrey's hand and injected a short acting anaesthetic. A push of the syringe, Jeffrey counts to ten, and slumps asleep when he reaches six.

The bronchoscope was inserted through Jeffrey's mouth and then pushed down through the larynx to the main airways. Pushing his bronchoscope through the larynx and into the trachea and main bronchi, the bronchoscopist had a view of the detailed anatomy of the airways. Thrusting down into the depths of Jeffrey's chest the bronchoscopist had sight of a tube of pink mucosa that evenly covered the ridges and runnels of the cartilage bands that supported Jeffrey's larynx and trachea. He moved further along the tunnel of Jeffrey's trachea, to the point where the trachea divides into two. This dividing point is called the carina. At the carina there is a fork where the right and left main bronchi branch off to the right and left lungs.

The bronchoscopist inserted his bronchoscope into the right main bronchus. And there, 1 cm away from the dividing point of the trachea, he saw Jeffrey's lung cancer, a bloody 4cm diameter cauliflower like growth.

He inserted a little brush into the bronchoscope and dusted the surface of Jeffrey's tumour with the brush. The brush was removed and its tip dipped into a specimen pot. Biopsy forceps were channelled into the bronchoscope and used to take a bite from the tumour. The bite was removed and placed in another specimen pot. The pots were taken to the pathology laboratories and Jeffrey was sent to the bronchoscopy recovery suite, a grand name for a small ward.

It takes a few days for the contents of the pots to be processed. The brushings were spun and the spinning process pools the cells taken from the surface of the tumour. The pooled deposit was smeared on to a slide, and then fixed onto that slide with a chemical dip. The smeared cells were then stained with dyes that made the architecture of the cells visible and interpretable.

The bite from the tumour was processed ending as a sandwich filler enclosed within a wax block. The wax block was fitted on to the arm of a lathe, and fine sections were cut from the block and layered onto slides. The shavings were fixed, stained and then examined under the microscope by a pathologist who comes to a view as to the precise nature of Jeffrey's tumour.

Lung cancers are divided into two main groups and these divisions, signal to the clinicians, pointers to treatment and prognosis. Lung cancers are classified as either small cell or non-small cell cancers. Small cell tumours are generally rapidly growing and at diagnosis have almost invariably spread microscopically to other parts of the body such as the bone marrow or adrenal glands. It is pointless operating on patients with small cell lung cancer because of this high chance of spread which means that any operation to remove the primary is of no benefit to the patient. Small cell lung cancer is generally treated with chemotherapy. The outlook for small cell lung cancer isn't that great, but nowadays more and more efforts are made to give multiple cycles of different courses of chemotherapy to most patients with this condition, because this class of tumour is so exquisitely responsive to treatment.

Non-small cell lung cancer is less likely to spread and can be treated by surgery or by radiotherapy given with curative intent. The outlook is much better than that for small cell lung cancer.

Jeffrey's case was to be reviewed in a meeting which gathered together doctors from many specialities. The meeting took about an hour and was held once a week in an ancient and musty, windowless and dusty lecture theatre. The meeting's purpose was to come to a consensus as to the management of the patients that were currently admitted to the wards. 'Cases' were presented and details reviewed. Conclusions were then drawn from the opinions of the team of doctors as to the best treatment for each of the patients presented. Serried ranks of doctors and medical students sat at stepped rows of tip up plywood desks and looked down on a pathologist and a radiologist who took centre stage in the pit of the lecture theatre behind an old fashioned teak surfaced desk.

The junior doctors took turns in presenting summaries of the patients' histories. X-rays were shown on back lit screens and the radiologist gave their conclusions as to the state of patients' primary and secondary tumours. Then the lights went down and microscope images of patients' tumours were projected on white screens for comment by the pathologist, who knows everything about everything, and accordingly gives his views.

Simon presented a summary of Jeffrey's history and the radiologist then put up his chest X-ray on the back lit viewing box.

"There is a right hilar mass, and it measures 6cm in diameter."

This from Dr Reznek a South African trained radiologist, a bright light of humour and intellect.

Dr Rose, consultant radiotherapist, a rather terse and humourless man who disliked Dr R's free spirit, barked from the front row,

"What's the lateral?"

By this was meant,

'What can be seen on the lateral X-ray view of the chest?'

To which came the slighting, exquisitely condescending, and wonderfully acerbic reply,

"It's an X-ray taken from the side of the patient, Dr Rose."

Every first year medical student, every junior nurse, would have known what a lateral X-ray was and this dry dust riposte was an immaculate put down.

And the hum of the whoosh of the collective sharp intake of breath from the assembled masses of doctors and medical students filled the room.

Dr Reznek filled the silence that followed the complete withdrawal of all of the oxygen from the room by a brilliant exposition of the changes shown on the lateral image of Jeffrey's chest X-ray.

The pathologist then topped up Dr Reznek's exposition with the light of his wisdom on the nature of Jeffrey's tumour.

"This is a poorly differentiated non-small cell lung cancer."

The doctors now knew Jeffrey's fate.

Their knowledge had an algorithmic path. Because the tumour was a non-small cell cancer, they knew that there were now options for Jeffrey's treatment and these were surgery or radiotherapy. Because it was poorly differentiated, meaning very rapidly dividing and dissimilar to the tissues from which it originated, they knew that survival chances were poorer than they would be for a well differentiated tumour.

The X-ray investigations had shown no sign of spread of the cancer so treatment could be given with curative rather than palliative intent. By curative intent is meant that attempts would be made to go all out for cure rather than treat merely to relieve symptoms.

But the bronchoscopy had shown that Jeffrey's tumour was very close to the point at which the trachea divided into the two main bronchi, the major tubes that take air into the right and left lungs. So close, that the thoracic surgeon would not be able to remove the tumour and close off the defect left in the trachea. The surgeon needs to be able to excise the tumour and a cuff of normal adjacent tissue in order to mini-mise the risk of the cancer recurring because of cells left behind at the edges of the cancer … and close the gap left when he has done his job. This was not possible for Jeffrey because of his tumour's location.

So what was left for Jeffrey as a treatment option?

Nervous Jeffrey could be treated with radiotherapy. The chance for cure with radiotherapy is less than for surgery and is about 15%. If surgery is technically possible then cure rates reach up to 70 to 80%. Radiotherapy treatment is now com-puter planned but in the early days of medicine it was not. The planning process then, was much more dependent on the individual skill of the treating radiotherapist whose expertise was used to define the areas of treatment. Now with com-puter imaging there is less 'subjectivity', and planning skills are based around the computer. With the aid of the screen we can see the borders of the tumour and map treatment dose around the geography of the cancer.

So an inoperable tumour … and radiotherapy was to be the next step on Jeffrey's road. Jeffrey's consultant, Dr Rose, gave him the news during the ward round, a procession of doctors and nurses around the in-patients. The conversation came halfway through the ward round, curtains drawn around

Jeffrey's bed in a parody of privacy, an environment that is exposed to the ears of every passing domestic, recuperating patient and inquisitive hospital visitor.

"OK doc."

The cascade of facial tics that normally crimped Jeffrey's face trickled to a halt. In this moment of the greatest anxiety, the torrent of nervousness that tormented his face was stilled by the kick of fate's bloody hammer.

"I'll go with that doc. Sounds all right to me. Didn't want them to cut me anyway. Me and my tumour … you know doc … we're OK together. We can live through it. He and me … well doc … we prefer being treated from the outside. Me and he … we'll feel better without holes."

So that was it. Jeffrey was going to have radiotherapy and that's how it was going to be for him. Treatment with radical intent. Downstairs to the toaster with him, the toaster, that's what the doctors called the radiotherapy machine. Once a day for four to six weeks depending on the treatment regimen used. All seemingly easy. Except towards the end of treatment when oesophagitis kicks in. The radiation umbra includes the edge of the oesophagus. This causes damage to the oesophagus. The lining of the oesophagus dies away with radiotherapy leaving the oesophagus red and raw. This can be unpleasant but it is easily treated with medicines that reduce the amount of acids in the stomach … a simple pill and potions that line the gullet and soothe away the pain. Oesphogitis is temporary; it comes towards the end of treatment and then fades away after a couple of weeks.

In the days when Jeffrey was ill, hospitals were for caring and not just for treating as they seem to be today. Patients were brought in to stay for the whole of their treatment period and in this way, the many possible side effects from treatment could be spotted and dealt with. Anything to get out of doing the dishes! Radiotherapy produces a tiredness that is cumulative, becoming more intense towards the end of a treatment program. So the patients could rest in hospital. Imagine such a thing in this current era! Nowadays the situation has changed, and there are many financial pressures to ensure that patients' residence in the wards is of minimal duration. It's cheaper treating outpatients, so treat them as outpatients ... and this is what doctors describe as the ASDA School of Medicine.

The treatment of non-small cell lung cancer has changed a little from Jeffrey's days. Doctors know now that some lung cancers, particularly those of unusual microscopic appearance and those affecting women, have proteins on their cell surfaces that recognise and bind to growth factors. Growth factors are proteins that stimulate cells to grow and divide. Too much growth and division are part of what makes a cancer. Some receptors, such as those for the epidermal growth factor can be targeted by treatment and turned off. This switch shuts down a ripple of molecular events in the cell, and when the ripple is switched off the cell dies. Drugs such as erlotonib target this cellular system and have been used successfully to treat some lung cancer variants, or rather ... treat some patients with lung cancer variants.

When they first were developed, drugs in this family of receptor blocking agents were thought to be massively important for many more than this narrow group of variant lung cancer. Drug trials in Japan appeared to be very significant and to presage enormous changes in the way that we would be treating lung cancer. The future had arrived and it was looking like targeted molecular therapies. The share prices of biotech companies soared and patients' hopes rose with the stock market. Unfortunately the story didn't pan out and the confirmatory trials brought negative results. However all was not lost ... except sadly, for the majority of lung cancer patients, because detailed analysis of the initial results showed that the responses to the miracle treatment had been in subgroups of patients, and these were women and patients with tumours of unusual subtype. For these patients the new treatments are of significant benefit.

So that's the targeted growth factor story, or a part of the story, but growth factor receptor inhibitors are not the only place where there have been advances in the treatment of patients with non-small cell lung cancer. We also know now that while chemotherapy has some benefit, the benefits are not great and so cancer doctors do not queue up in a great rush to offer their patients treatment with chemotherapy.

The weeks went by as they do if you are lucky, and as they also do when you are unlucky and Jeffery, well Jeffrey was in the camp of the not too unlucky... but only in that not too unlucky camp for a while.

Three months from the completion of radiotherapy the march of Jeffrey's time tramped to another camp where there was trouble brewing in the cooking pot.

One of the registrars phoned Dr Green from the out patients clinic. The call was from a man whose career advancement had certainly benefitted from his rugby skills. Tom would never even have got into medical school if he hadn't been 6 feet 7 inches tall when he was 17 years old. Tom, if he hadn't weighed 220 pounds, would never have passed his college exams. Tom, a man who was not failed simply because he was so bady needed in the medical school rugby team, a man whose patients certainly had no gain from his killer strength in the scrum.

"Can you book him in?"

No please. No background information, just the order to book him in.

Poor Jeffrey had been pushed to the ward in a wheel chair, and was waiting in the reception area for a bed to become available on the ward. Poor Jeffrey! He was in a state.

"What's happened Jeffrey?" Dr Green asked.

Half of Jeffrey's face looked as though it had slipped off his skull. The left side of his face hung loose, and when he tried to speak his cheek blew out with the effort. His left arm hung lose and useless. His left, slipperless foot had fallen from the footrest of his wheelchair.

"Just came on doc.

"Don't know how doc.

"Over a couple of weeks. Gradual, you know what I mean doc, then boom."

Jeffrey's cheek bulged with the boom.

"Look at me doc!

"Not going to win prizes at the baby show, am I doc?"

And spittle dribbled down his chin.

When a patient with cancer has symptoms such as Jeffrey's, the doctor's initial diagnosis is deeply gloomy, and it is that the patient has had spread of his cancer to his brain.

Cancer spreads either through the lymph system or through the bloodstream. Single cells break away from the site of the primary tumour, and fleeing away in a tidal stream of blood or lymphatic fluid, travel to distant parts of the body. These single cells end their journey trapped in terminal networks of small blood vessels, like a shrimp washed up on a beach by the breaking waves, trapped in a web of tangled seaweed.

The journey ends for these cells in the capillary networks of organs with good blood supplies, ends in the lungs, bones, liver or brain. In these distant capillary jungles, the cancer cells take nourishment from the nutrients carried in lymph or blood, and grow and then divide, grow again and divide again until the tiny clumps of cancer cells have become bigger clumps, and have become of sufficient size to cause a problem to the organ in which they have nested. In the liver, the cancer cells can cause jaundice by physically damming the drainage of bile. In the lung, the metastases can cause breathlessness and in the brain …

The cancer prevents the brain functioning and the particular loss of function depends upon the site of the spread of the cancer. Different parts of the brain have different roles, controlling the way we hear and see, move and think. All of these functions have complex cerebral regulatory pathways and the regulation of function is undertaken through neural lines that funnel through many levels of the brain. In Jeffrey's case the cancer could be pressing on one or possibly more than one of a number of points where the brain controlled movement.

The diagnosis of where precisely in the brain the metastases sat is made by clinical assessment and judgements are followed by scans to confirm or refute the provisional diagnosis. Diagnoses mainly come from the patient's story, are confirmed by examination and refined by scans and X-rays.

The most important clues come from the story. It's very rare that for the experienced doctor anything is added by examination findings.

An initial conversation with Jeffrey had given all of the clues needed to make a diagnosis. Jeffrey had explained that his weakness had come on gradually over a couple of weeks, and the doctors clearly knew that he had cancer. So because lung cancer does have such a high chance of spreading to distant sites, it didn't take an Einstein to make the connection. However, there are other causes of loss of power in your limbs, and the most important is stroke, caused by bleeding or a blood clot. But strokes are usually rapid in onset and often accompanied by acute headache. Jeffrey's symptoms had come on slowly and this is much more typical of cancer spread than stroke.

For a moment Dr Green's doctor patter stumbled to a halt. He felt that his questions seemed so pointless. Dr Green looked at Jeffrey, slumped in his wheelchair, pale and poorly, unknowing of his fate. He saw what would unfold for him over the next few weeks and felt ... well felt pity for him. What had he had in his life, what joy, what gifts, what hope, what strength? Marginalised, as 'Subnormal', never a job, never a wife nor children, anxious, at the fringe, never at the centre of society, peripheral, at home with his mum, and now this. Dr Green reached out and gripped Jeffrey's forearm, touched the softness of his egg and dandruff scarred cardigan, felt the warmth of him and he looked up, puzzled at the contact.

It was likely that Jeffrey had a secondary cancer growing in the motor cortex on the right side of his brain, a hypothesis that would be proven by a brain scan. He was admitted to the ward with that working diagnosis, bloods were taken, and a chest X-ray booked to re-assess his primary lung cancer. The doctors wanted to see whether or not it had grown back, and understand from his blood tests if there was evidence of any changes to other organs such as his liver. The bloods and the initial X-ray were done on the day of Jeffrey's admission, and the results were normal, but they had to wait a couple of days for there to be space in the scan list for Jeffery. And while the doctors waited, the medical students gawped.

The scan confirmed the clinical diagnosis, but not only was there a secondary in the motor cortex but, as is typical of lung cancer, other secondary cancers could be seen too. The images that the doctors peer at on a light box in the X-ray department are portraits of Jeffrey brain printed on A4 sheets of negatives. These pictures portray the brain as a rather large grey, black and white walnut, sliced horizontally. The brain usually appears symmetric, but for Jeffrey the beautiful grey shaded symmetry of the cortex and other brain structures is perturbated by darker dysmorphic shadows where the cancer sits. Little black pebbles can be made out in the light grey of Jeffrey's motor cortex, pebbles with varied density and ragged edges.

The radiologist shakes his head as he looks at Jeffrey's scans. He shakes his head, his predominant thought that Jeffrey's fate could be his fate. He knew that he really, really … must stop tipping off and having those sneaky fags in the gap between barium enemas, because there is no way that he wanted to be Jeffrey.

The doctors started treating Jeffrey with steroids. There are all sorts of steroids, some steroids make you beautiful, some steroids give you muscle, some produce facial hair and some put fat in all the wrong places. But the steroids that we give to cancer patients don't make you beautiful. They make your face puff up and they weaken your muscles. They give you indigestion and they can make you diabetic, they disturb your sleep and lead to mood change.

But hey … for all this, they can make you better.

For all of the downside there is an upside. Doctors haven't taken all those years to train to cause misery; they have trained, believe it or not, to make patients better.

Steroids act to reduce the swelling and inflammation around a tumour. A large part of the changes that could be seen on Jeffrey's scan are caused by swelling and inflammation. Often doctors will give a trial of steroids before radiotherapy treatments commences to see if there is any improvement in the patient's neurological function. If there is improvement then radiotherapy is given because that magical improvement with steroids is indicative of a high chance of a response to radiotherapy treatment. If there is no gain with steroids then the 'pain' of radiotherapy is avoided because treatment with radiotherapy is unlikely to produce an improvement if steroids have not helped the patient. In this situation radiotherapy treatment can be avoided and usually is. This is because cerebral radiotherapy can cause sickness and fatigue, nausea and hair loss, all side effects of treatment that need to be bypassed if there is going to be no benefit in terms of improved neurological function and increased life span.

After a day or so of steroid treatment Jeffrey picked up. His face resumed its usual contours and he was able to walk with a Zimmer frame.

Hunched over his frame, he looked up at Dr Green as he walked into the ward.

"I'm not for the Olympics doc."

"Were you a player Jeffrey?"

"In my day doc! In my day! I was faster than anyone on Dalston Lane. And when it came to giving the shopkeepers the slip ... I was the boy."

"Is shoplifting an Olympic sport Jeffrey?"

"Doc ... In the right circumstances it can be."

So, improved a little by steroids, Jeffrey took another trip to the basement for radiotherapy treatment and with the passing of a few days he became stronger and stronger and made it home eventually to the care of his good old mum, care, unfortunately that didn't have long to run.

That was non-small cell lung cancer, and now we move on to small cell lung cancer, which is not at all like its cousin. Amazing how the absence of three lower case letters and a hyphen makes such a difference to a disease. But there again the word 'cancer' is almost malign itself in the confusion that it inspires. 'Cancer' is such an elision of bewilderment, such a concatenation of confusion. The generic 'cancer', describes and binds together a large and immensely varied family of diseases with exquisitely different manifestations, kindred of enormously varied significance, vastly diverse treatments, and hugely dissimilar outlooks. The term 'cancer', is a conspiracy of the malign to confuse and confound. Cancer may not need to be treated, might need to be treated or might not even be worth treating depending, just depending on its site of origin, microscopic appearance and extent of spread.

Small cell lung cancer is not the most cheerful of diseases to treat, but treat is what you usually need to do.

Ron is lying exhausted, sleeping in bed in the ward. He had straight black, slicked back hair but that's long gone now, long gone with the first round of chemotherapy that he went through. He's a tall, thin man in his late 50s. Ron was a used car salesman with his own showroom in the Hackney Road. He specialised in high end cars, the Mercedes and Jaguars, BMWs and Range Rovers, the species of motor appreciated by certain groups of East London people, the men with bulging pockets, the folks who did deals for cash. Cash rich, cheque poor, invoice free, that was how the business was run. Ron had a lot of help in the business from his family. There was Carol his wife, blonde but basically brunette, Carol did the books and Angie his daughter, more blonde than blonde, was front office. And then there was Dean his son, a chip off the block, and there had been many chipped blocks in the process of manufacturing Dean.

Carol and Angie and Dean stood around Ron's bed looking away from him. They watched the ward and the ward watched them. The ward seemed to be waiting for something to happen to Ron and Ron's family were waiting for something to happen to the ward, anything but to share Ron's state.

Ron had been through three different interludes of chemotherapy treatment. He had gone through a long, tough 12 months. His time had been marked by periods in which he had symptoms, periods when the symptoms resolved because of treatment and periods when the ordeal of treatment had been almost worse than the symptoms of his cancer. Three different treatment programs had been given to him at each point in his illness when his symptoms had progressed.

Ron had been a heavy smoker; like so many smokers he had started burning the evil weed when he was 12, cadging smokes of friends and nicking boxes of ten from his dad's top shelf. Ron had got up to 20 a day by the time that he had left school at 15. He'd stopped smoking the moment that he started to cough up blood, thought he had better stop before it was too late, but by the time that he started to think that he better pack in the fags it was of course 40 years too late to stop smoking. One of the signs that tell a doctor that something serious is wrong is when a patient reports feeling out of sorts and then adds that,

'You'll be pleased with me doc, I've packed in the fags.'

The doctor is not all pleased that his patient has shoved his fags in the bin. He knows that the cessation of smoking by a middle aged man is virtually diagnostic of mortal illness, and is ironically, rather sorry that his patient has given up smoking.

Ron had no qualifications when he left school, but he did have had gold starred certificates in charm and humour. He had started trading on a market stall in Petticoat Lane, helping out a friend of his father. Ron was as sharp as a dodgy pair of stilettos. He'd gone on to have his own stall, then a shop and had traded cars on the side. The car business worked for him, worked big time. It was amazing what a good wipe down with T-cut could do for the sale price of a motor. And the judicious application of T-cut shone the way to possession of the car showroom.

Ron's coughing blood had led to X-rays, the X-rays had led to outpatient appointments, the outpatient appointments had been followed by bronchoscopies and biopsies and multidisciplinary review and multidisciplinary review had been followed by referral to an oncologist.

The oncologist was Dr Healey, formerly of High Wycombe, a pipe smoking man, small and perfectly formed, a smiling man, with a fine collection of double breasted waistcoats, and watch chains, vestiges of his grandfather's fashion sense, vestiges that worked particularly well for him.

Dr Healey seemed to saunter on ward rounds, a little out of focus with the ethic of work, taking his time to appreciate the nurses, taking so much time to appreciate the nurses that he would often seem to lose the thread of the discussion and have to be re-orientated by his registrar.

Dr Healey was loved, because in his heart there was kindness, and empathy. He knew how the patients felt and he knew what motivated his juniors. He was laconic and inspirational, but he did get distracted whenever there was sight of a pretty face.

But back to Ron. Ron had been given chemotherapy when he first came to the attention of the cancer specialists. At the beginning, although all of the staging tests had shown no spread of his cancer, the presumption was that as the cancer was a small cell variant there would be evidence of spread, by the very fact that it was a small cell cancer. Small cell lung cancer grows rapidly and spreads very early in its natural history. So when the primary tumour is small even smaller sites of secondary spread will already have been established. Now scans and X-ray have their limits, and one of their major limits in defining the extent of tumour spread is their ability to register small abnormalities in internal body organs. Changes are only visible on conventional X-rays and scans when the size of the abnormality measures over 1 cm in diameter.

Furthermore, the imaging tools that we have, the ultrasound scans, CT scans, and MRIs, can only show the doctors changes in the anatomy of internal organs. They do not allow the clinicians to have a microscopic view of the patients' internal structures, nor do they allow us to come to a view of the way that those structures are functioning. We look at shapes outlined in shades of grey and en grisaille gives no clues as to microscopic detail.

This failing has been partly addressed by the development of PET scanning. PET scanning gives clues as to the functional activity of internal organs. One of the most commonly applied PET scanning techniques is called FDG PET. FDG PET enables us to have an idea of the metabolic activity of internal organs. Cancer is generally more metabolically active, and requires more sugar as a fuel, than normal body organs. This need for sugar is exploited in PET scanning. A radioisotope is attached chemically to a glucose molecule and injected into the patient. The radioisotope collects preferentially in the cancer which is more avid for sugar than normal tissue. The radiation energy emitted from the sites of uptake of the radiolabelled glucose can be measured and those measurements used to provide a Google Street Map of cancer location. But even with this tool we cannot define the extent of small cell lung cancer spread to distant organs from the primary site, because the sites of spread are microscopic and do not collect enough radioactive glucose to register on a PET scan.

Studies of patients with small cell cancer who have died at an early stage of their illness have shown that early spread is ubiquitous and inevitable. Not only are the scans which have been incapable of showing small deposits of secondary cancer useless, but even worse ... results in small cell lung cancer give a false assurance of normality. Microscopic analysis at post mortem of organs that appear normal shows the invasion of cancer cells.

As a result of this evidence we know that systemic rather than local treatment is required for small cell lung cancer, however small the primary appears to be. Radiation and surgery only treat part of the cancer; they are focussed treatments. As it's not possible to sterilise or cut out enormous numbers of microscopic metastases there is no real point to surgery or radiation given with curative intent.

So chemotherapy is given at an early point in the careers of lung cancer patients. It's the Heineken approach that's needed. Something is required that will reach all parts of the body. And that something is chemotherapy.

Chemotherapy for small cell lung cancer collects together groups of drugs that have a wide variety of mechanisms of action. These include a group of drugs called alkylating agents. For a cell to divide, the DNA needs to make a replica of itself, but it cannot do this if the two strands cannot come apart, so when a cell is treated with an alkylating agent it cannot divide.

Ron had been treated with these drugs, had been re-treated, and then had gone on to receive further chemotherapy. This had been given by mouth and for Ron it had seemed initially that the pill had been a whole lot easier than treatment with intravenous chemotherapy. But he had been deceived by the ease with which the tablets had slipped down.

Ron sat in the outpatient clinic consulting room and explained his views on this outrageous deception to Dr Healey. As Ron confided his views to him, Dr Healey gazed wistfully out of the grime smudged window at a group of first year nurses walking across the grass in the sunshine. In the consulting room a tap bled into a cracked sink. The clinic room clock had stopped last winter. The clinic was in the basement of the building and so it was important that Dr Healey concentrated on the view, for here in the basement there were the benefits of an angled vision, from below to above, from his creaking desk chair to pleasant parts, to the lower regions of passing strangers, and as Dr Healey knew only too well, to the passing parts of people that he knew.

"You know it's a real bugger Dr Healey, 'scuse my language. Slips down easy with a sip of water, and you think, 'cos it don't make you sick, that you'll be fine.

"Not so doc. No way will you be fine. It slips down and next thing you know, the very next orf, bam, your gone, you're in 'ospital with bleedin' infections."

"Quite so."

Dr Healey patted his waistcoat pocket and crossed his legs.

'Blast!' he thought 'Where have I put my pipe?'

"Dr Healey, as I was saying, it's a killer it is. Tablets down your gob and then next thing you know you're in an 'ospital bed with a drip in your arm and antibiotics shuffling in like they love you.

"Dr Healey. You think you're going to be OK 'cos five days later you're over the infection and in the Range Rover driving 'ome with the lovin' family.

"Sure, you're 'ome with the loved ones but ... next thing ... you're waking up come the morning, scratching your 'ead, wondering what's for breakfast and you notice that it's your skull you're scratching and that you've left all you 'air on the bleedin' pillah."

Dr Healey had completely lost the thread of the conversation, so taken was he with a particularly pleasant view of the scenery, a view that took in a vista of the delicate contours of knickerless youth.

Ron, sensing that he was not the object of Dr Healey's full attention, coughed.

At the cough, Dr Healey's gaze flicked back into the room, and the owner of the gaze, attention lagging a little behind his eyes, noticed for the first time in about three minutes that he was not alone in the room. With a start, Dr Healey focused on the patient, his patient, Ron.

"Beg p-p-pardon." he stammered.

And Ron quite misunderstanding the apology, continued

"Sorry Doctor Healey, my language, she's always on at me, she is. Sorry."

"Not at all, you were saying ..."

But Ron had quite forgotten what he was saying and so the conversation shuffled to a halt with gifts of blood sample forms from Dr H to Ron.

But that was three months ago and now Ron was in the ward, his family in attendance, and Ron was sick. Since the conversation with Dr Healey he had had another three months of chemotherapy treatment. He had taken the little pills for seven consecutive days and these treatment days had been followed by 21 days off treatment. This 28 day period constituted a treatment cycle and each had been complicated by an admission to hospital with one side effect of treatment or another. On one occasion it had been an awfully sore mouth, on another bad constipation and the third admission had been because of infection.

So Ron had had a rotten time. Quality of life? Not great. And now ...

'Poor Carol …' thought Ron, from the tumbling depths of opiate dreams

' … She has to see me like this.'

And this … this was a seven stone man, the skin of his bottom broken by a bedsore, a bald man, nursed on a ripple mattress, a man stuffed with morphine, a man needing help to turn in the bed. No wonder the family faced out from his bed, looking at the passing world and not wanting to witness his pain. And pain. Ron did have pain. It was his thigh. Hurt like Hell, or rather as he said in a hoarse, spittle thickened whisper …

"Urts like 'ell."

But then, there seemed to be an odd distraction to his statement. It was as if he was describing an event that involved a third person, something was happening, but happening to someone else. Dr Healey had looked after a man who had been a Second World War hero. He'd commanded a warship and his boat had been sunk in the North Sea. He lasted 16 hours in the freezing water and was rescued. Amazing luck because of the fact of his rescue, and also because of the 'other' fact of the extraordinary miracle of his survival for so long in the water. Most normal people last 12 minutes in the cold of the North Sea, and at the end of those minutes their heart stops from hypothermia. There was clearly something different about our hero's heart and our man went on to become Britain's ambassador to a Far Eastern country. In retirement he developed lung cancer and the cancer spread. The cancer gave him pain, but as he said, in the last few days of his life,

"It doesn't matter, strange thing, the pain is there but I am here, it's almost as if the pain is an irrelevance. And as to the pain killing tablets … you know, I take the pain killers and the essence of the pain isn't really altered by the tablets. They do have a strange effect. They change my perception of the significance of the pain. The pain remains, but the tablets seem to have made the pain matter even less than it did. "

And so it seemed to be with Ron. He was describing pain in his thigh, but that pain seemed to be affecting another person.

"Best have it X-rayed Ron."

An exhausted Ron, family in attendance, went for an X-ray. He was taken to the X-ray department in a trolley as he was too sick to walk, too sick even to sit up to be pushed over to the X-ray department in a wheelchair.

Ron's X-ray showed him to have a large metastasis in the head of his thigh bone. Healthy bone looks on X-ray like a pipe that's been cut through longitudinally. The walls of the pipe, the cortex of bone, are thick and white against a background of black. At the top of Ron's femur there were the beginnings of a large crack. The bone at that point was grey and not white, and the grey area was where the bone had been thinned by spread of his lung cancer. This was a metastasis and Ron's femur had been weakened by this spread. The lung cancer cells had travelled in the blood from Ron's lung and lodged in the bone. There, plugged into a little hiding place in Ron's femur, taking nourishment from the ample supply of blood that bathed the bone, the lung cancer cells had divided to form a mass of cells that had disrupted and damaged the normal structure of the femur. The hard material that makes up bone had been replaced by soft cancer cells, chalk had become cheese, and the cancer cells that had no substance, cancer cells that had no had no structure, took away from the strength of Ron's femur.

Ron had pain in his leg and the cause of this pain might at first seem hard to understand. Bone itself has no pain nerve supply but the periosteum, which lines the surface of the bone, does have pain sensing nerves. A metastasis raises the periosteum and by doing so leads to the release of pain provoking chemicals. Many of the drugs that control pain do so by blocking the effect of these chemicals on pain sensing cells.

Dr Healey was called to the ward by his registrar to look at Ron's X-rays. It is usual for consultants to come on ward rounds at fixed times. Ward rounds are an event of high ceremony and drama, a parade of doctors and nurses held twice weekly at most. But such was the urgency of Ron's situation that the registrar had felt it important to break with routine. Dr Healey, his juniors and the nurses gathered around the

X-ray and at that point Dr Healey's great humanity, a humanity that eclipsed his foibles, radiated through.

"Poor chap.

"Best get an orthopaedic opinion and see what can be done …

"Let me talk to him."

The curtains were drawn around Ron's bed and the family gathered around. Dr Healey sat on the edge of Ron's bed, sat close to him, legs crossed and Ron gazed up at him from the pillow. Dr Healey looked around at the gathered ward round and said,

"Best be off chaps, I'm sure that you've things to do."

The doctors and nurses busied themselves with tasks, but remained within distance of the bed, distanced, but close enough to hear the conversation. The experience that the juniors gain from their apprenticeships in medicine comes like this sometimes, comes from behind drawn curtains, and the experience marks doctors' lives and redefines their behaviour.

The juniors were witnesses to conversations, observers of humanity, passively listening to what sometimes must be said.

"So Ron, how are you feeling?"

It was very unusual for Dr Healey to address his patients by their first name. By using Ron's first name he was telling him that this was a special conversation and that he had a personalised and special feeling for him. And it was clear that he did have a special feeling for Ron.

The gathered doctors could hear Ron mutter,

"Well doc …"

"How do you think you're getting on?"

This is an open ended question that allows the patient to tell the doctor their thoughts. Some patients will turn the question back to their doctors, hoping or not hoping for information depending on the tone and emphasis of their response. Others will say in a noncommittal way that they are 'OK', really asking for confirmation that they are OK and some will say as Ron said,

"Doc, I'm fucked …"

Now doctors are taught to respond to this sort of statement by asking why the patient feels that he is stuffed, but Dr Healey, bless him, did not do text books and said,

"Ron, I think that things are a bit tricky …

"But we can help you so don't give up. Ron, we have a plan."

Although they couldn't see him the doctors knew that at that point in the conversation Dr Healey had laid his hand on Ron's arm, and by his touch given Ron strength. Dr Healey understood, as a result of his life's experience with cancer patients, that what Ron needed was not the sourness of truth, what Ron needed was hope. It is very much against the teaching of modern medicine to be economical with the truth. Doctors are taught that truth is the property of the patient. The patient must be in possession of the facts and the patient must decide for himself what to do with those facts.

But what is the kindness in telling a man or woman that they will be dead in a day or two, where is the humanity in taking away all comfort, why is there a need to deny all hope?

Dr Healey had told Ron that there was still something that he could do for him. And that is the truth because there is always something that can be done, pain can be eased, breathlessness helped, constipation dealt with. Something can always be done, even in the dying moments, an unpleasant cough can be cured, or a sore mouth calmed. Something can always be done. Dr Healey had told Ron that there were options because his sense of Ron was that Ron needed something, Ron needed something to hang on to, all hopes could not be dashed.

But if Ron had said to Dr Healey,

'I am not dying, am I Dr Healey?'

What is it that Dr Healey should have said in reply?

Again there may be a sub-text to the question, sub-textual implications that depend upon the tenor of the question and rely for its answer upon knowledge of the man.

This sort of question does require probing before it can be answered properly. In some contexts the patient will want to know the whole truth about their situation, they might wish to say things to his friends and loved ones that must be said, they might need to make financial arrangements, they might have a truth to tell.

In this situation doctors are taught to ask why the patient thinks that he is dying. This allows the doctor to understand what it is that the patient wishes to know and what it is that a patient is frightened of. For some it is fear of the unknown. Will death be painful, will death be terrifying? There are many stories of patients who have been resuscitated, snatched from the jaws of death and brought back to life. These patients always tell tales of enveloping peace and the brightness of unbearable light, they describe overwhelming joy, tell of comfort and immense peace. So although one can never really know what death is like, it is likely that the march to death isn't unpleasant. Either there is a God or the flood of endogenous endorphins that mark any traumatic life event are sufficient to …

And Dr Healey knew his man.

The orthopaedic opinion was called up and the orthopods clumped along to Ron's bedside. They scratched their heads as they stared at Ron's X-ray films and concluded in whispered conversations, in the recesses of the wards, that he really was too poorly to stand an operation. Ron would not make it through the anaesthetic. It was their opinion that Ron was at such a risk of dying from the anaesthetic itself that it could not be justified offering him a place at the operating table.

So where next? How would the doctors deal with Ron and what would they say to Ron's family?

The curtains drawn, Dr Healey told Ron that he would treat his leg with radiotherapy. Radiotherapy is an excellent way of treating pain, but it can weaken bones.

The nurses were very keen that Ron's family were asked what their views were on cardiac resuscitation. There is a uniform policy in all hospitals that all sick patients are either asked personally for their opinion about cardiac resuscitation, or in the event that the patient is too poorly to have that conversation, then a family member is asked what their view is about resuscitation. By this is meant they are asked what they feel about the nurses calling the cardiac arrest team if their relative's heart stops on the ward. By 'heart stopping' … is meant 'dies'.

Now death is inevitable, inescapable, and the ubiquitous fate of all humanity. For a cancer patient, although the odds are good for survival, death comes to some. When death comes rattling at the doors of the ward, all the body systems pack up, the lungs fail, kidneys and liver pack their bags, the peripheral circulation gives up and with a gentle sigh, another soul leaves the planet. That the heart stops at the end of this process of organ meltdown is almost an irrelevance. For dying patients with cancer any attempt to restart the heart is futile. Imagine a loved one dying at the end of a long period of illness, family gathered round. The arrest team is called and efforts are made to re-start the cancer patient's heart. The body is engulfed by a battalion of doctors and nurses, drips are put up, defibrillators applied and the corpse 'shocked', attempts are made at cardiac massage, an airway is inserted and then after 15 minutes of panic and drama, dignity of death in a cleaner's bucket, the squad gives up because the cancer patient has died, from cancer.

Studies have been carried out in which the survival rate of patients dying from cancer who have had a cardiac arrest call out have been investigated. The failure rate of the resuscitation attempt is 100% and the success rate, to labour the point is 0%. In contrast, in the situation when a cancer patient who is not dying from cancer, has a cardiac arrest, the chance of successful resuscitation is exactly the same as that of a patient without malignancy. The cancer patient's chance of survival is the identical to that for a man or woman who is in hospital with appendicitis or pneumonia; the success rate is about 30 to 40%.

In other words, when a patient is dying of cancer any attempt at cardiac resuscitation is absolutely futile. Furthermore, any discussion about a patient's wishes in this situation will cause the patient distress and make the patient's relatives think that they are empowered or burdened with the gift of life or death, and that their decision is vital in determining outcomes.

The application of a blanket policy in hospitals, where all patients are asked what their views are … is an emotional disaster. Why ask, why raise hopes, that Mum or Dad could be brought back from the dead, when they cannot. Why raise the prospect of the assault of the cardiac arrest team summoned by a shrill bleep from the depths of the hospital, when resuscitation is worthless for the terminally ill cancer patient and the outcome is entirely predictable? But on UK wards the doctors are made to be agents of policy that is pointless, policy that causes distress, policy that makes people think that death can be survived, when it cannot be countered.

Ron's treatment with radiotherapy started the next day, and he went down to the radiotherapy machines to begin a treatment program that was scheduled to be completed in five days. About 80% of all cancer pain is relieved by radiotherapy, but the painkilling effects of radiotherapy treatment usually take up to two weeks to kick in. In the meantime, waiting on the ease of pain, Ron's painkilling tablet dosages were increased, and they needed to be increased on a twice daily basis in order to keep his pain under control.

Dr H was very involved in Ron's care. He came to the ward twice a day to see how he was getting on and took time from his schedule to talk with Carol and the children. They, rather than Ron were keepers of information, because Ron was too ill, and too numbed by morphine to have much of an idea as to what was really going on.

Dr H had made the judgement, understanding his man, that Ron didn't need to know any more. Ron, he judged, had had enough news to keep him going, but for the rest of the family the situation was different: they needed to know. It is hard for a family to have more insight than the patient. It drives division and wedges, makes it difficult for there to be communication, but in some situations secrets are needed.

Carol was sitting with Dr Healey in the nurses' office. Her roots were showing kohl black, but although she was looking exhausted her makeup was just sublime. She had a nice line in turquoise eye shadow and her foundation spoke of sunrise to sunset suntans made in Mauritius.

Dr Healey leaned towards her and crossed his legs.

"How are we all doing?"

Carol gave no answer.

Carol cried quietly and long lines of mascara traced down her cheeks and spotted her blouse.

Dr Healey reached for the tissues and passed her the box.

"He's looking very poorly.

"I think you need to be prepared for the worst ..."

Carol sniffed, blew her nose loudly and then nodded her head.

"I don't think it will be long. Sorry ..."

"I know. But it's so hard to just sit there and watch him like this ..."

"Yes, it is just ghastly."

Dr Healey reached over and stroked her shoulder, then stood up and walked from the nurses' office. As anyone could see who would look, Dr H's eyes had reddened, only a bit, mind, only a bit. Sometimes it's difficult for the doctors too.

It was Friday afternoon and Ron had just been brought back from radiotherapy. Dr Green watched as the nurses began to turn him in the bed trying to avoid yet more bed-sores, doing their best to make him comfortable. Ron was tipped gently onto his side, one nurse supporting him from behind a second nurse standing on the opposite side of the bed holding Ron, one hand on his hip, another on his shoulder pulling Ron gently towards her, and ...

"**AAAAAAAAAAAAHHHHHHHHHHHHHHHHH**."

Ron howled. His scream seared the ward. He roared in agony. The nurses were transfixed, horrified. The patients stared, all sat straight in bed riveted by his pain.

Dr Healey rushed to Ron's bed. Ron's back was arched, and his hands were clasped around his thigh. Ron's face was contorted with pain. He held himself rigid. His leg was bizarrely angulated, as if put on the wrong way round. It was clear to

Dr Healey what had happened. Ron had fractured his femur through the metastasis. The weakened bone had snapped.

Ron's eyes were clamped tight. Tears trickled down his face. His mouth was open. His chin was pushed out from his face. His neck muscles were rigid. He was panting, he was sweating.

The nurses gathered round.

"Morphine please, sister."

And a syringe and vial appeared. The nurses rushed to pull the curtains together. The hushed and horrified and the merely curious were shut out. Ron juddered with pain.

The nurses steadied Ron's arm and Dr Healey found a vein. The morphine was injected in a rush and in a few seconds Ron's body became limp and he was unconscious. Ron's breath came evenly and his arms fell away from his leg.

"Strapping please, sister …"

Dr Healey wrapped thick white adhesive plaster around Ron's thigh. As he worked he took care to concentrate on Ron's face, stopping his work if the movement of Ron's leg caused pain, stopping to inject more morphine to keep Ron unconscious. The strapping was attached to weights hung from a little pulley at the end of Ron's bed. The effect of the strapping and weights was to keep Ron's leg under tension, the strapping kept taut so that the femur was fixed and the pain of movement was minimised.

"Can you call Carol in please?"

And one of the nurses went to call Carol.

Dr Healey sat with Carol, Angie and Dean and the Macmillan nurses. He explained what had happened and told them that Ron's time was now very short.

"You'd best tell the family …"

"But they're miles away …"

"Look, tell them all, but see if you can designate somebody to make the calls. Let them know Ron's really poorly and then it's their decision alone if they want to come or not. Because afterwards …"

And Dr Healey's voice tapered off. His hesitation was deliberate, almost theatric, and the meaning of that hesitation was,

'There will be no recrimination from family members who didn't choose to come along to pay their last respects.'

A morphine pump had been set up. The pump was a grey box measuring six inches long, an inch deep and two inches wide. It cradled a syringe clasped within the embrace of two elastic bands. A clear tube led from the syringe to a tiny hollow needle embedded in the skin of Ron's tummy. There was morphine in the syringe together with an additional drug given to stop the nausea caused by morphine. The pump pushed slowly on the syringe delivering a steady infusion of drugs to Ron, drugs to keep him comfortable.

Ron did look at ease, at peace, his breath quiet.

"Carol, his time has come. Our efforts now are to keep him comfortable …"

"I understand Dr Healey. There is no future for him. There is no point in him suffering any more. It's enough."

"The pump … it doesn't hasten him on his way."

There is a space in time for every person when every thing is suspended, and for Carol, that moment had come. And in that moment all movement in the ward ceased and the silence was deep. All was in freeze frame, every nurse every patient, every doctor every cleaner, the phlebotomist and the medical students, the porters and the visitors. The bustle of life died and the phones stopped ringing. Light faded and the fog of quiet came rolling around. Then sight was returned, a great boom of ambient sound flooded, then roared and time resumed its bitter song.

Carol looked up and Dr Healey was there.

'I am here and he is there. Ron is over there and I am here. But why, why …?'

A jumble of entirely coherent illogical thought rushed in and out of Carol's mind and all that she really knew was that her life was over.

'And Ron, poor Ron …'

The family gathered, came and went, brought food for Carol, food that was left in the corner of the single bedded side room to which Ron had been moved. As patients and visitors walked past the door to Ron's room it seemed as if their pace slowed, as if they were caught in the magnetic field of the drama, clasped by arms reaching out from a life ebbing to its end. As each person approached, the weight of their footsteps increased, knowing that Ron's passing signalled their passing, the inevitability that all spirit must fade.

The nurses had put in place the Liverpool Care Pathway. The Pathway formalises and regulates the medical and nursing care of the dying, allowing patterns of care to be put in place that maximises the comfort of the dying. Some doctors and nurses will argue that the Pathway makes dying into a process, an inexorable process, with rules and regulations, makes dying formulaic. Many doctors and nurses dislike the Liverpool Care Pathway because of its rigidity but the Pathway's proponents argue that it is not a rigid way of caring for the death but rather a way of death that ensures the maximal attention to the patient's needs, ensuring that mouth care, pain control, bowel and bladder care are all of the highest quality.

It used to be that if a patient was thought to be dying of cancer, that his end was hastened, minimising pain by doubling the morphine dose every two hours. This approach still has its advocates but is not practised because it is considered both immoral and illegal. Some years ago a case was brought against a doctor. Some of the close family of a dying patient had asked the doctor to help their dying family member who they thought was suffering inordinately. The doctor, seeing the terminal nature of the cancer patient's illness, had taken it as his responsibility to inject potassium, which caused the patient's heart to stop.

However, other family members had been horrified by his action and had taken the doctor to court. The judge ruled 'manslaughter'. In his judgement, the judge gave the opinion that if a drug is given with the express purpose of ending life then the intent is to kill, and that could not be countenanced. But the judge, in what is thought by the medical community to be an entirely wise addendum to his ruling, went on to state that if a patient died as an indirect consequence of a drug given to ease symptoms such as pain then the doctor would be acting entirely within the frame of the Law.

A drip was put up to provide fluid. This was done to give Ron comfort and not to medicalise the process of dying. It is thought, with absolute evidence, that dehydration is uncomfortable and so fluid replacement provides ease to the final days.

Ron had been catheterised because a full bladder is painful, and the catheter had been put in place for this reason, and not as is sometimes thought by relatives, to make the job of the nurses easier.

Every hour the nurses came in to swab Ron's mouth with a pink sponge lollipop drenched in water. A dry mouth is really uncomfortable and the swabbing moistened his mouth.

Ron's breathing became harsh, rasping and irregular. His breath rattled and became coarse and sticky. The nurses added a new drug to the pump. The new drug dried the secretions in his lungs that were the cause of his noisy breathing.

Dr Healey popped his face around the door frame, hand clasping the door, not stepping over the threshold, he asked,

"How's it going, are you all right, is there anything that we can do?"

It was as if he was embarrassed by the vacuity of his questions, and didn't want to encroach on the privacy of the family in Ron's dying hours. But of course he was wrong, he was loved and the family was grateful to him for coming to the ward.

"Talk to him, hold his hand, somewhere he'll know you're all there. Tell him about when you met. Tell him you'll be all right, tell him if you can bear it, talk to him if you can manage it."

In the depths of death there is comfort to talk, it's a diversion, it helps. And it is thought that it is a support to the dying, because amidst the fog of death the clouds are swept away for moments by lucidity, and comfort comes from knowing that you are not alone. But this is a hard call on the family.

Dr Healey left the family and as he walked the corridor of the wards, as he passed the nurses' station, a great wailing caught his ears, a primitive lowing and howling that rushed at him and took away all breath.

Chapter 5
Conference With Counsel

"Everyone here?"

This from the barrister's clerk, a tall man, stooped and edentulous, his bleak and cadaverous form draped in a grimy suit. The clerk rubbed his hands together, and balancing on one foot and then another, surreptitiously shined the tips of his shoes on his socks as he addressed the group of five people assembled in the waiting room of counsel's chambers. The group sat on lumpy armchairs covered in pale blue Draylon, sat around a glass topped coffee table laden with grubby copies of *Country Life* and *Horse and Hound*. Who was in the waiting room? There was John Crowe, a solicitor, Henry Green a GP, Doctor Rosenberg an oncologist, Professor Sleight a pathologist, and Sylvia Hitchings, widow of Alex, around whose case the conference with counsel had been scheduled.

The experts had come together to discuss the details of Alex's case in order to prepare for the next steps in the process of litigation.

"Mr Armitage-Shanks will see you now. Would you like to follow me gents into the conference room please?"

And ignoring the fact that the clerk had disregarded her presence, chin held high, Sylvia led the group, and the clerk, into the conference room. The conference room looked over the gardens of the Temple. There were modern prints on the walls, images of lavender fields in Provence, bought as a job lot on eBay. Glass fronted bookcases lined the room, filled with dusty enfilades of leather bound copies of law reports from the last century. Through narrow windows there were views of flickering sunlight on the grass slopes leading down to the Embankment.

The barrister rose to greet his visitors. He was, as all barristers should surely be, dressed in a pinstripe double breasted suit, cut away collar, club tie. There is no credibility to the words of a barrister who has no striped suit. As he stood up a flop of hair fell untidily over his forehead and he swept the hair away to a flash of dazzling cuff and heavy gold links.

"How do you do everyone, do please sit where you'd like to ... sit

"Professor please do sit ...

"Mrs Hitchings ..."

And with a generous gesture of his hand that took in the room, its prints, the bookcases and the view, the barrister showed his visitors to their places around a conference table.

Everyone in their place, the barrister set the scene.

"Now, Mrs Hitchings, we will be speaking of matters that I'm sure will make us appear insensitive and for this please do forgive us. Do you see ... the purpose of this conference is to determine whether or not we can proceed in law, and the basis for proceeding is the strength of the case ...

" ... Mrs Hitchings ..."

And the barrister paused to pass his fingers through that elegant flop of hair that had fallen again, but in a dammed attractive way, he thought, over the elegant heights of his forehead.

"Mrs Hitchings, do you see ... what we have to prove ... is that on the balance of probabilities ... your late husband would have survived if there had been an early diagnosis of cancer ..."

The barrister warmed to his theme and turned to the solicitor to brief him on the points of law that had to be dealt with. Now Mr Crowe had an entirely satisfactory understanding of the law in this matter but was sufficiently cowed by the hectoring manner of the barrister to be taken back to patterns of behaviour that had evolved in him during his hard years at public school, taken back to the ingrained lessons of life that came from the rule of class, size and aggression that had dominated his school days.

So Mr Crowe, in his tweed jacket, clutched at his black Samsonite briefcase, found a pen and paper and wrote notes in red biro on an A4 lined pad, as he listened to the barrister's waffle.

The barrister continued …

"And not only do we have to prove … Mrs Hitchings, do you see … that the doctors who were involved in your late husband's case were negligent in their management of his symptoms but we also have to prove that your late husband would have survived if an early diagnosis had been made.

"So, there are two tests that we have to pass in order for there to be a chance of success in this case. We have to prove negligence and we have to show causation.

Mrs Hitchings crossed her legs and straightened her back. She undid the top two buttons of her powder blue cashmere cardigan and leant forward, concentrating on the barrister's words.

'This case!' she thought.

'He means Alex. Alex wasn't a case …'

"There is a test, do you see … that we have to apply … to the doctors. This is called the Bolam test. The Bolam test has to be passed in order for there to be a chance of successful litigation. We have to show that the doctor's management fell below a standard that would have been considered acceptable by the doctor's peers. In other words we have to prove, do you see, that the GP practice was of a poor standard. This is the Bolam test … it is a test of negligence, do you see?

"And this is where our first expert witness comes in to play.

"Now gentlemen you will have before you an agenda and a chronology that I have prepared for the meeting. You do have the agenda? John you have distributed the papers?"

The barrister turned to Mr Crowe inquisitorially.

There was silence as the group focussed upon Mr Crowe who had clearly not distributed any papers.

"Not to worry, here they are. I had brought along an additional set in the event of failure."

The barrister stood up and doled out stapled papers to the group. Everybody except Mrs Hitchings was given a copy of the barrister's agenda and chronology of events.

'I'm not important enough to have my own papers!' thought Mrs Hitchings.

But then Dr Green, sitting next to her said,

"Why don't you share my papers?"

And pushed the barrister's agenda and chronology towards her.

There was a sharp rap at the conference room door and the barrister's clerk bustled in.

"Teas, coffees anyone?"

The order was taken and the clerk shuffled out. The conference room door closed and the barrister turned to Dr Green.

"Let's concentrate now if you would on my chronology. I'd like to go through the sequence of events and understand if I might, what should and should not have happened following each of Mr Hitchings attendances at the GP's practice."

Alex's story had started five years ago. Sylvia remembered so clearly how it all had begun. Alex had gone to his GP; he'd been made to go by Sylvia after she'd walked into the bathroom to sort out her makeup and found blood in the lavatory pan. She had noticed that he'd been constipated recently and that was unusual for him, he was so regular a man in all his ways, bless him.

"What's this?" she'd called to him.

"There's blood in the pan … what's going on?"

"I'm not sure, it just came. Maybe it's piles or something?"

"You've never had piles before. You better go along to the GP and get sorted out. Maybe he'll give you something for them …"

"I'll be all right, it'll sort out. I'll wait and see and if it happens again then I'll go along. Don't want to bother him with trivia!"

"No. Don't wait. That's just like you to leave things. Where has waiting ever gotten anyone anywhere …?

"Leaving things! Go along and get yourself sorted out. I'll ring up for you and make the appointment."

Sylvia was brought back from her memories by the boom of the barrister's voice, brought back from distant days that seemed in her mind to be so vivid, so close in time, brought back to the gathering of medical and legal opinions at the conference table.

"Now Dr Green, I would like you to consider, if you would, Mr Hitchings' first visit to his GP's practice."

Dr Green pulled out his reading glasses from the top pocket of his jacket where they nestled behind a folded paisley handkerchief, and peering through thick lenses, scrabbled through the bundle of photocopied notes in a grey plastic bound A4 folder that lay on the table in front of him. He searched through the records to come to a rest at the point in the GP's computerised practice records that described Mr Hitchings' visit to the practice with symptoms that marked the first presentation of his illness.

"Aahh …" said Dr Green,

"Here it is."

"What does it say?" asked the barrister.

Dr Green peered at the notes with quizzical concentration and then pronounced,

"This is what the GP has written …

"Rectal bleeding for two weeks. Small amounts of bright blood on tip of stool. Constipated recently.

"And then …" Dr Green took off his glasses to rub his eyes and then putting his glasses back on read,

"R J, Anusol."

"And what does R J mean Dr Green?"

"It means Recipe of Jupiter!"

"What!"

"Yes recipe of Jupiter. That's what older doctors were taught to write as a short hand for 'prescription'. It's a vestige from history, left over from a time where the gods were invoked for the cure of disease."

"Hmm, very interesting, but not at all relevant Dr Green. Let us keep to the point, do you see. Anusol?"

"It's a common over the counter medicine for piles. It acts as a local anaesthetic and soothes your tail."

Professor Sleight, the pathologist, considered the consequences of the anatomical aspects of the concept of the tail and was rather amused.

"Concentrating, Dr Green on the matter in hand, if you would, what do you think, Dr Green, of the standard of Mr Hitchings' GP's conduct at this initial consultation?"

Dr Green removed his glasses again and looked up at the barrister.

"It is an understandable approach but it is not good practice."

"Why, Dr Green, why?"

"Because the GP should really have examined Mr Hitchings, and then referred him on for a hospital specialist opinion."

"So was it poor practice to have not done so?"

"I believe it was."

"Do go on ..."

"You see, new rectal bleeding in a middle aged person must always be taken seriously. It is indicative of serious pathology unless ..."

The door to the conference room swung open without a warning knock and the barrister's clerk entered bearing a tray laden with cups and saucers, coffee and tea.

"I'll leave it here, gents, for you to 'elp yourselves if you would. Mind the coffees is very 'ot. Don't go scalding yourselves dears, mind yourselves."

And out flounced the clerk, having changed, the pathologist noticed, into an evil looking pair of monogrammed suede slippers. Professor Sleight wondered if the clerk shared the slippers with the barrister and giggled to himself.

"Shall I pour?" asked John Crowe, eyes widening at the prospect of Jammie Dodgers.

"If you must. Now, can we please concentrate on the matter in hand?" exclaimed the barrister.

"Dr Green, consider if you would, the standard of medicine of an average GP? Did Mr Hitchings' GP's standard fall below that average standard on the occasion of this visit to his clinic?"

"Yes, I believe that it did."

"Perhaps you would be so good as to tell us in what way the GP fell below the standard?"

"Certainly. It is mandatory on a GP to follow through on a story of rectal bleeding. He didn't respond appropriately to Mr Hitchings' history of constipation. The GP should have asked Mr Hitchings if he'd had any family history of bowel problems and then gone on to examine his patient. And by examine is meant both an abdominal and a rectal examination."

"Mrs Hitchings …?"

And the barrister nodded at Mrs Hitchings who was just bursting to interrupt, but in contrast with the barrister's clerk, Mrs Hitchings waited for permission to interrupt. It was not that Mrs Hitchings had coffee to serve. It was simply that Mrs Hitchings was far too polite to follow the clerk's example, and furthermore she had absolutely no wish to share the clerk's slippers. Mrs Hitchings said,

"It's funny that you should mention Alex's family history and his bowels. His father and a cousin died of bowel cancer, and I was always going on at him to have some testing done … And he had become constipated, always off round the Chemists getting some potion or other to help him go, beggin' your pardon."

"Would it have been appropriate for Mr Hitchings to have had any pre-emptive testing?" asked the barrister, turning to Dr Rosenberg.

Dr Rosenberg had been sitting quietly throughout the proceedings. He'd been day dreaming, thinking about his kids and how the medico legal conference, would, if he was lucky, and it went on for long enough, increase his income by about £600 which would cover one sixth of one term's school fees, for one of the kids, or rather he continued to muse, one-twelfth of the fees after tax, or one twenty-fourth of both the kids' fees after tax.

Dr Rosenberg folded his musings into his empty wallet and attended to the barrister's question.

"Pre-emptive testing. Screening is what we call that," he mumbled, gathering time to orientate himself into the conference proceedings.

"The current national policies on screening for bowel cancer are not great, bit of a dog's dinner actually.

"How do we screen? In the first instance as an initial screen, a normal adult can have their stools tested for blood. This involves them putting a small sample of their poo, as we doctors call it …"

Dr Rosenberg paused for a laugh but then, realising that he had completely miscalculated the mood of his audience, coughed into his handkerchief and continued,

" … onto a piece of paper. The paper is sent off to the labs and subjected to a chemical test for blood. If blood is found then the normal person becomes a patient and is recalled for further tests, such as a colonoscopy … but this is not the best way of screening for bowel cancer."

"Why?"

"Because the test is very sensitive and picks up benign and very common causes of rectal bleeding like piles. As a result, a lot of people are frightened into thinking that they might have cancer and end up having a lot of unnecessary further tests."

"Is there a better test?"

"Better? … Yes.

"Better is a colonoscopy, done every ten years from the age of 50. You see, bowel cancer grows very slowly, accumulating a rolling snowball of molecular changes that make it more and more malignant. The cancer starts by showing changes in the genes of a few cells. The genetic changes grant longevity to the cells and as a result they divide, grow and become a larger mass of cells, clumping together, expanding, until with time they appear like an abnormal growth of tissue, what we call a polyp.

"Then further molecular changes are acquired, and the polyp subtly alters and takes on more overtly malignant features. The polyp invades the lining of the bowel, invading more and more deeply, until finally cells break off and spread into the lymph and blood systems and showers of seedling cells are dispatched like triffids to distant parts of the body.

"If you can get the polyp at an early stage in its career, then you can stop its development and halt the procession of events that end with malignancy. Colonoscopy is the polyp's career stopper.

" … The doctor looking through the eyepiece of the colonoscope, searching along the pink tunnel of bowel, can spot polyps as they rear up in his sights. The polyps wave at him and he waves back, waves with biopsy forceps, snags the polyp with his forceps, and clears them from the bowel aborting their growth before they've had a chance to get to the malignant stage.

"Put simply, the colonoscopist aims to abort the baby polyp, and once in the bin that terrible baby will have lost the chance of growing up to be a big boy cancer. In other words a screening colonoscopy will stop the inexorable development of bowel cancer at an early stage, and halt its growth at a point when the polyp is still harmless."

For a moment, he dwelt in his mind on the exquisite sequence of molecular events that unravelled in the development of bowel cancer, a march of mutations that had been elucidated by a saxophone playing scientist who had gone on to receive the Nobel Prize for medicine. The Nobel for medicine … it wasn't like the Peace Prize, the winner deserved it, he thought.

Mrs Hitchings burst in on his revelry.

"But why doesn't everyone have a colonoscopy?"

Dr Rosenberg turned to her.

"Mrs Hitchings … it's because a colonoscopy is expensive. It's just not possible for everyone in the whole country to have this procedure."

The barrister didn't like the way the discussion was evolving. They were all going off on a tangent. He was in charge and he'd let them all know it.

"Turning now to the point, Dr Green." interrupted the barrister.

'That would show them!' he thought,

'Tell them all who's boss.'

"You say that the GP should have examined Mr Hitchings as well as take a proper history. What would he have been likely to have found if he had examined Mr Hitchings?"

"He may have found nothing and strangely that's an important observation, or he may have found blood on the finger of his glove when he carried out a rectal examination."

"May we deal with each of those points?"

'They would be dealing with these points,' the barrister thought.

'There was no question of any dissidence. They were only doctors, and they would be answering his questions in the order that he posed them.'

"Now Dr Green. Pleased do tell us why the absence of any sign was important."

"It would have told the GP that Mr Hitchings obviously did not have piles as a cause for the rectal bleeding."

"And the blood on the glove Dr Green?"

"That would have confirmed Mr Hitchings' story and shown that there was a significant cause for the bleeding."

"And reverting to points about medical standards … was the failure to carry out this assessment negligent?"

"I believe so, but the answer to your question is a little complex. May I explain?"

The barrister nodded Dr Green on,

"Very well, if you must."

"You see, strangely enough, it is not mandatory to investigate a single episode of rectal bleeding. So Mr Hitchings' GP does not fall below the standard on the basis of ignoring the single attendance at his surgery. Research has shown that a single episode of bleeding is not diagnostic of a sinister pathology. So, on some counts, and I say some counts, advisedly, it would have been reasonable at this point merely to have asked to review Mr Hitchings again after a couple of weeks.

"Why do I say this?"

The barrister had no idea why Dr Green had the impertinence to raise a point without proper consideration.

"I say this because the average GP is tasked to be informed about current practice and this includes him being aware of government guidelines.

"You see, there are government guidelines that have been laid down to assist the GP. These describe and define indications for referral for many conditions. The current guidelines for the investigation of rectal bleeding would not have suggested to Mr Hitchings' GP, if he had bothered to read the guidelines, that he would have needed to have referred Mr Hitchings to hospital for a colonoscopy or to see a gastroenterologist.

"However, in a way, that's an irrelevance because Mr Hitchings also had constipation and referral is mandatory for a patient with rectal bleeding associated with a change in bowel habit.

"The GP certainly should have taken a proper history. The family history of bowel cancer, bleeding and the change in bowel habit are critically important features."

At this point in Dr Green's discourse, the barrister had become clearly irritated with the doctor. It was Dr Green's role to answer his questions succinctly. This rambling discourse could not be tolerated, blast him; blast him for the lower middle class softy that he was, a socialist too, no doubt.

"So ... " he interrupted, raising his voice,

"Was Mr Hitchings' GP negligent at that point? Should he have referred him for assessment?"

"Yes. I believe that his practice was negligent, as I have written in my report."

"Bolam negligent?"

The barrister had risen to his feet. It was as if he had imagined himself in court interrogating his witness, in front of milord the judge.

Mrs Hitchings had also risen to her feet, taken with the emotion of the awfulness of her loss and the culpable negligence of her husband's GP. Her hand went to her mouth and she flushed.

At the same moment, Mrs Hitchings and the barrister noticed that they had got up from their seats and resumed their places.

"Can you explain if you would, doctor, about the significance of the family history of bowel cancer?"

There was something so deeply patronising about the way that the barrister had said the word 'doctor'.

"Well I would if I could …" Dr Green replied,

"But perhaps one of the other experts could chip in?"

The barrister glowered at Dr Green who, in his mind, had an improper lack of deference to the fact that he was in charge of the proceedings and that therefore it was up to him, the barrister, to make the judgement call as to who should deal with what. The conference was to his mind getting out of hand and he didn't like that for one little moment.

'For goodness sake!' he thought,

'It's not as if any one of the lot of them had been to Eton and who, may I ask, amongst them read Classics at Magdalene?'

"Perhaps I can help," added the pathologist.

The barrister nodded.

"If you would please professor."

"A small proportion of patients with bowel cancer have genetic conditions that predispose them to the cancer. These conditions, and there are several, are inherited. Mr Hitchings' family history suggests that he might indeed have had one of those conditions, and for this reason, the GP should have been alerted to the fact and ready to make a referral. I believe this to be the case from my reading of the guidelines."

'Bloody pathologists,' thought Dr Rosenberg,

'What is that they say? … the pathologist who knows everything but knows it too late, the physician who knows everything but does nothing and the surgeon who knows nothing and does everything!'

"So, Dr Green, we conclude that the GP was negligent in not examining Mr Hitchings and also in failing to refer him on for either a colonoscopy or for a hospital appointment.

"Now, let us examine, if you would, the other areas of negligent GP practice. Help us, please, Mrs Hitchings with this Please do tell us what happened after Mr Hitchings' first appointment?"

"Well, Alex was reassured by his visit. He thought there was nothing wrong, poor man. Little did he know! He popped along to the chemists and bought himself some really strong laxatives. Didn't tell me about it mind, never grumbled, never complained, bless him, just took the medicines. I only found out months later, when I cleaned out the bathroom cabinet.

"So then I said to him, I said, 'Alex, you're to get along to the doctors again, you shouldn't be constipated at your age, there must be something wrong,' I told him, and then I said again 'Alex, go and get it sorted out.' I remember it as if it were yesterday.

"Well, I went on and on at him, poor man, and in the end he did go along to see the doctor again.

"I went with him to the surgery. Well, he spent about two minutes with the doctor and then he was sent out of the room with a flea in his ear, as if he'd done wrong in bothering the doctor with his trouble."

"Dr Green, is there any evidence for this consultation in the contemporaneous medical records?"

Dr Green peered into the records and said,

"Yes ... there's a consultation on the 18th July and the only entry in the records on this occasion is 'Piles again ... R J Anusol, again."

"And your view about negligence."

"It is my view that the GP was negligent, negligent again."

"Do please go on, Mrs Hitchings."

"Well, poor Alex was getting no better at all. In fact, he was getting worse if anything, poor love. So ..."

And Mrs Hitchings paused to dab at the corner of her eyes with a screwed up lace handkerchief, pulled from the sleeve of her cardigan.

"So, Mrs Hitchings, so ..."

Mrs Hitchings straightened herself up and replaced her handkerchief in her sleeve.

"Yes. So ... Alex went again to the doctors again. And he told him again that he was very constipated and was passing blood."

"Dr Green, can you confirm?"

And Dr Green, quite the barrister's puppy said,

"Yes, it's here in the notes, 14th October, 'constipated …' he writes … 'Rectal bleeding … 'Try Movicol.'"

"Movicol, Dr Green?"

"It's a laxative."

"Negligent again, Dr Green?"

There seemed to be a glimmer in Dr Green's eyes as he answered,

"Who me? I hope not!"

The barrister was not amused and drummed his fingers on the conference table.

"Negligent, would you say, Dr Green?"

Dr Green coughed and answered,

"Yes. Certainly."

"And what should have happened on this occasion?"

"In my view, as what should have happened on all the other visits to the GP practice, with symptoms of rectal bleeding and altered bowel habit."

"Yes, Dr Green …"

"Mr Hitchings should have been referred for a colonoscopy or for a gastroenterology outpatient appointment."

"And Bolam negligent at each visit?

"Yes."

"Would you like to tell us, Dr Green, if you would, how many visits there were with these symptoms?"

It didn't seem as though the question from the barrister gave Dr Green the option of not describing the visits.

Dr Green rustled through the notes and said …

"There were visits to the GP with similar symptoms on the 26th November, 17th December and then, in the following year, on the 2nd and 28th of January, 3rd February, 16th April, 27th July, and then there's a gap …"

"Yes!" exclaimed Mrs Hitchings.

"There was a gap because, as Alex said, there didn't seem to be any point at all in going to see the GP, as the GP never got things better. Alex said … that it would just have to be something that he lived with, but …"

And her voice trailed off, as she looked out with reddening eyes over the splendid lawns.

'It's time for that wretched handkerchief again!' thought the barrister.

'Really! Quite extraordinary! Don't these people know how to behave?'

"Ah, I see, do carry on, Mrs Hitchings."

"Well he went again to the GP and again, even though he didn't think that there was any point in going. He went because I nagged him to go. I wish that I'd nagged him to go and see another doctor. We should have gone private."

'Bloody woman!' thought the barrister.

'No reason to become emotional. Why can't she focus?

'Focus woman for goodness sake!'

"Dr Green, your view, please."

"From the GP's notes, one can see that there were further visits with similar symptoms on the 12th September, 19th October, 22nd and 23rd of November and then into the following year on the 13th January, and the 12th and 16th March."

"And then …?"

"And then Mr Hitchings is seen on the 1st April … but by a different GP."

'The blighter gets lucky at last!' thought the barrister.

"By a locum. And the locum recognises the significance of Mr Hitchings' symptoms and makes a referral to hospital. And he does so under the two week wait cancer referral guidelines."

"Meaning?"

"That the GP suspects a cancer diagnosis, and accordingly the hospital appointment has to be issued by the hospital, for a clinic date no less than two weeks after the receipt of the GP's referral letter."

"So, why might we ask was this referral not made at any of Mr Hitchings' other GP appointments? Why is it that Mr Hitchings' original GP failed to make an appointment for him to be seen at the hospital?"

"It's not clear why. Sometimes of course the GP has just got the wrong end of the stick and made an incorrect diagnosis. It happens. A diagnosis in medicine is not always based on absolutes, there is a deal of skill, and subjectivity, sometimes doctors just get it wrong because they have made the wrong call in the beginning and haven't seen any reason to change that call."

'Wrong call!' thought Dr Rosenberg, 'Wrong call indeed.'

"So, to summarise," boomed the barrister,

"There has been a delay of about 18 months in referral and that delay is without doubt negligent.

"Over to you now, Dr Rosenberg. Can you help us now with the hospital side of things?"

'No please … not me, I hate the arrogance of that man, and he's picking on me now.' thought Dr Rosenberg.

"So, Mr Hitchings is seen in outpatients on the 14th April. The registrar seeing him, notes his history and writes in the records,

'History of rectal bleeding for 18 months.'

"He observes that Mr Hitchings has a family history of colorectal cancer. He then goes on to examine Mr Hitchings, and when he carries out the rectal examination, describes finding blood on his glove."

"Go on, Dr Rosenberg, do go on."

The barrister appeared as though he were conducting an orchestra of experts, waving one doctor in and another out, pronto legalto.

"The registrar arranges for Mr Hitchings to have blood tests, a chest X-ray, and a colonoscopy."

"The colonoscopy is booked for a week following the out-patient visit."

"Is that a reasonable interval from the outpatient appointment?"

This enquiry from Mr Crowe was an interruption that he felt important to undertaken in order to remind everyone in the room that not only was he actually in the room, but that he was also a lawyer, and not only was he actually in the room and a lawyer, but that he had also organised the conference. But his interruption merely served to startle everyone, merely served to surprise everyone with his forgotten presence and furthermore irritated the barrister, who after all, was in charge of all legal proceedings, and indeed, in charge of all life itself.

And the intensity of the negative energy emanating from the barrister focused on this worm of a legal being, sucked all energy sources from the room and dimmed the conference room lights.

The solicitor's extreme temerity in interrupting the sequence of questioning was a profound and base example of lèse-majesté, in the view of the barrister.

"May I remind everyone that it is best, do you see, that we have one person in charge of the conference, otherwise time will be wasted, no doubt, on irrelevancies, and that person in charge should, according to protocol, be the barrister. Me."

"Dr Rosenberg, is that a reasonable interval from the out-patient appointment?"

"Yes."

"Good. Now, do go on Dr Rosenberg, do tell us what happened next to Mr Hitchings?"

'*Chrrrrist*, that man is just awful.' thought Dr Rosenberg,

'Wonder if he lines up his wife and kids for a kit inspection before they leave for school in the mornings?'

"Well, the colonoscopy took place sure enough, but no cause for the bleeding was found ..." continued Dr Rosenberg.

"Yes, Dr Rosenberg. Proceed."

"And Mr Hitchings was seen in clinic after the colonoscopy and given a six month appointment for review."

"Is that a correct course of action, Dr Rosenberg?"

Mrs Hitchings could stand it no longer; she'd been bursting to comment.

"No, of course it wasn't right ... poor Alex, he was losing blood each day, I fed him steak to keep his strength up ... and ... and ...

And Mrs Hitchings' voice tailed away to a noisome silence as her handkerchief emerged from the puff of her sleeve.

"... It wasn't right."

"Could you explain why it wasn't right, Dr Rosenberg? Could the Court know why it wasn't ... to use Mrs Hitchings' word ..."

'The Court!' thought the barrister, distracted by the sound of those two beautiful words, his words,

'The Court!'

And the barrister's words seemed to tail off for a moment. Discourse halted, he appeared to be disorientated for a moment, lost to the conference, lost in dreams of a seat at the Court of Appeal to which he had aspirations.

"It wasn't right, your honour ..." said Dr Rosenberg,

'Who's a cheeky boy?' he thought,

'Hope I got away with that?'

Everyone except the barrister had spotted the faux pas.

"It wasn't right because the colonoscopy had not been a thorough and complete assessment."

Mrs Hitchings took a sharp breath in and touched her fingers to her lips.

"If you look at the record ..."

Dr Rosenberg pushed forward the folder of Mr Hitchings' hospital notes to show the barrister. and Mr Crowe, the record of the colonoscopy.

The legal beagles scrutinised the colonoscopy record which showed that the examination had been incomplete. The barrister sat reading in full and comfortable view of the records, while the solicitor stood at an awkward angle, peering over his shoulder. The colonoscopist had written,

'Incomplete assessment. Poor patient preparation. Suggest repeat after good bowel preparation.'

"If you look at the notes you will see that the colonoscopy had only gone from the anus to the splenic flexure, gone to the point where the bowel turns a corner. At that point, his view obscured by faeces, the colonoscopist had aborted the procedure. And this is vital ... thus aborted, Mr Hitchings' transverse colon and ascending colon hadn't been visualised. In other words only half the large intestine had been looked at.

"Now you should know that I give my view as a consultant oncologist and gastroenterology is not my specialisation. It may be that Mr Crowe will seek the opinion of a gastroenterology expert witness to examine this matter of gastroenterology negligence in more detail."

Mr Crowe beamed.

'What a nice chap!' he thought.

'We'll use him again. What about that Morecombe case? I'm sure we'll need an oncology opinion there. Jolly good chap.'

"I don't think so, Dr Rosenberg. I am not sure that we will follow your suggestion. I will not advise the Court that we require an additional medical opinion, do you see.

"But pray, do continue. Do tell us what should have transpired, do say."

"Mr Hitchings should have had the procedure re-ordered. Better laxatives should have been prescribed to Mr Hitchings so that his entire bowel was cleared out and the bowel lining could be properly seen. The repeat colonoscopy should have been carried out within two to four weeks of the failed procedure."

"And did this happen?"

"Unfortunately not."

'Unfortunately …' thought the barrister.

'Certainly not! Unfortunately! I think not! Poor choice of word. Fortunate more like, otherwise we wouldn't have a case, and I wouldn't be sitting here.'

"Go on, Dr Rosenberg."

"Well, six months later …

"Oh how that poor man suffered." sighed Mrs Hitchings.

"Six months later, Mr Hitchings pitched up to clinic and saw the consultant. A second colonoscopy was booked with good bowel preparation beforehand and, lo and behold, there, bang in the middle of the mid transverse colon, in full view, was a large, friable …"

Mrs Hitchings' sniffed …

"Friable in this context means brittle to touch, bleeding when prodded by the colonoscope."

"Thank you doctor."

"The tumour was biopsied and Mr Hitchings was seen with the biopsy results two weeks after the colonoscopy."

"Go on doctor, proceed if you will."

"Yes, his case had in the meantime been reviewed at the multidisciplinary team meeting. You can see the notes of the meeting on page 332 of the records. The pathology report had shown Mr Hitchings to have a moderately differentiated adenocarcinoma and a provisional plan was put in place for Mr Hitchings to have a surgical clinic review. But before the surgical outpatient appointment, the meeting had concluded that the diagnosis should be conveyed to Mr Hitchings in the gastroenterology outpatient clinic."

"Is that what happened Mrs Hitchings? Did you go to the gastroenterology clinic first?"

"No, we didn't, we went straight to the surgeon. The gastro-enterology secretary phoned us and said that the clinic was overbooked, and so would we mind if they speeded things up by sending us straight to the surgical clinic. Well, of course I didn't mind … anything to get poor Alex sorted out.

"That was a terrible experience, mind. The surgeon, bald chap with a bit of a tummy, he didn't introduce himself, just came in the room and said,

'I agree, it needs to come out, we'll have you in and sort everything out for you. The juniors will book you in,'

"And then he said, and I remember it so clearly,

'Next patient sister, where are we going? Where are you taking me next? Paris, I hope! Jolly good!'

"And then he laughed.

"But the appointment did turn out all right in the end …

"Because this lovely young doctor came in, and found me weepy. She was ever so pretty, Natalie, that was her name, lovely manner, blue eyes and black hair. She told us why Alex needed an operation, explained the procedure, and then said she was very sorry the surgeon had upset us but we weren't to worry because, although he wasn't too good with people, he was extremely good at his job. She arranged a scan for Alex, a CT scan."

The barrister had had enough of Mrs Hitchings.

'Time to move on.' he thought,

'Time to get to the nitty gritty.'

"Dr Rosenberg. Can you help us please? What happened next?"

"Surgery."

"Thank you Dr Rosenberg. Anything else that you would wish to add?"

"At operation they found a very large primary tumour and …"

"Yes Dr Rosenberg …"

"And also found, that unfortunately, there was extensive spread of the primary to the liver."

"Yes …"

"Too extensive to resect. You see, the operation had proceeded on the basis that they knew from the scans that Mr Hitchings' cancer had spread to the liver. So they had planned a combined approach that involved a colorectal surgeon and a liver surgeon. However, when they opened his belly …

Mrs Hitchings gasped.

"Sorry, Mrs Hitchings."

"Please go on doctor, don't mind me."

"You see, they had found that Mr Hitchings' tumour had spread so extensively to the liver that any attempt at hepatic resection would have proven impossible."

"Why, pray?"

"Quite simply, there was more tumour in the liver than normal tissue. Just impossible."

"But why, Sir, would they have wished to chop out bits of the liver?"

"An attempt is made to resect the secondaries, because if resection is possible then the chance of Mr Hitchings surviving is significantly increased. The surgery is pretty extensive, but the benefits are also extensive."

"I see. But they couldn't?"

"No. Technically, as they say, impossible."

"Go on, Dr Rosenberg."

"So, as we know, Mr Hitchings went on to have chemotherapy. Got better for a few months, went on to have more chemotherapy, relapsed again and then was treated with a new biological agent. Got better again."

"Can you tell us a little, Dr Rosenberg, about the treatment of colon cancer with chemotherapy? I need to understand the treatment and understand also about the symptoms that Mr Hitchings is likely to have had, so that we can put in a claim for 'Pain and Suffering'. You know of course that pain and suffering has a distinct financial value to our client?"

"Certainly. Colorectal cancer treatment has advanced considerably over the last few years. We have many new treatments, some of which are chemotherapy drugs and some of which are the new generation of medicines, the biological agents.

"The chemotherapy is relatively mild in terms of side effects, sore mouths, diarrhoea, sore chaffed fingers and toes are the main problems that treatment causes to the patient."

"Oh yes, Alex had those all right. Had them by the bucket load!"

"And the biological agents work by targeting receptors on the surface of the cancer cells, receptors made by the activated oncogenes in the cancer. They are only present in a proportion of patients."

"I don't think that we need to go into that sort of detail, do you see. Do stick to the point Dr Rosenberg, there's a good chap."

"I am sticking to the point, as you will see if you would let me answer your question …"

The barrister glared at Dr Rosenberg.

"If I may continue? The receptors, if they are present in the tumour, are also present on normal skin and bowel cells … so the targeting is to these normal receptors as well as to those on the tumour. As a result patients can get skin rashes and diarrhoea as a side effect of treatment with these new classes of drugs."

"Oh yes, Alex got them all right, got them awful."

"And one might expect if a patient is responding to these new agents that he's very likely to look as though he's reverted to adolescence, with spots and reddening of his face."

"But all these drugs … how do they help the patient? We've looked at their downside but how do they impact upon the patient's life?"

"They achieve a lot. They impact significantly. The survival of patients with metastatic colorectal cancer has increased from about nine months to two and a half years, with some patients surviving five years or more, nowadays. That increased longevity is down to the new drugs. But there is a cost to consider. It's estimated that the cost of treating a patient with metastatic colorectal cancer, the price of the drugs alone, is about £250,000. So if you think about the cost of the disease to the nation ..."

"Dr Rosenberg, you may finish now. Thank you, we now know all that we need to know from you for the purposes of this conference. You are dismissed. Thank you, though, for your help. Most kind. Good day."

The barrister stood to point Dr Rosenberg to the door, and the good doctor, aghast at the barrister's coruscating manners, shuffled his papers together, shook hands with his colleagues, Mrs Hitchings and the solicitor, and left the room, passing out from counsel's chambers.

The door closed and the barrister turned to interrogate the pathologist.

"Professor Sleight. Over to you now.

"You are, I believe, a pathologist, and quite eminent in your field. Is that correct?"

"Quite eminent? I think that it is for others to judge my eminence or lack of eminence."

"Perhaps, but it is I who am asking the questions. Are you considered to be eminent in your field?"

Dr Green answered for Professor Sleight.

"He is a world expert. He taught me pathology when I was a student. He wrote the textbooks that we used at medical school."

"Thank you, Dr Green. Now professor ... now that I understand that you are reasonably well considered amongst your colleagues, we can turn to the pathology findings. Professor, can you explain to us what the pathology findings were? Could you enlighten us, professor?"

Professor Sleight's hackles had risen to ceiling height but he did his best not to be supercilious in his answer, tempted as he was, to let the barrister know that enlightenment was not his profession, but was the empire of priests and other charlatans.

"I have examined the tumour and support the original pathologist in his description of a moderately differentiated T4 colonic cancer."

"Meaning, Professor Sleight? Meaning?"

"Meaning that the tumour appears to be of moderate grade and advanced stage."

"Help us, please. Grade? Stage?"

"Grade is the appearance of the tumour under the microscope. Grade ranges from relatively benign, which is described as well differentiated, to nasty, which we call poorly differentiated. T stage is the extent of spread of the tumour, and T4 indicates that the tumour has spread from the colon to surrounding tissues."

Professor Sleight recalled a time some years ago spent in court explaining to the judge the difference between stage and grade. The judge had had great difficulty in distinguishing between stage and grade, and had been inordinately confused for the duration of the trial about the differences between the two terms.

"Yes, so Mr Hitchings had a G2 meaning grade, T4 N2 … meaning stage …

"N2?"

"N describes the extent of spread to the lymph nodes draining the tumour."

"Ah, and Mr Hitchings' had spread?"

"Yes. He did have spread to the nodes."

"I see."

"And he also had spread of the tumour to his liver. Extensive spread as we have heard."

"Now, gentlemen!"

'That's it,' thought Mrs Hitchings.

'What is it about counsel's chambers that they classify all human beings as male? There they go … ignoring me again!'

"Gentlemen, we have clearly shown negligence in Mr Hitchings' management. We have shown absolutely and unequivocally that there has been a delay in the diagnosis and the treatment of his condition and we turn now to the issue of causation.

"Mr Crowe, this is, as you know, the crucial aspect to the case. We, as lawyers, have to show that there has been a loss of chance as a result of the negligence, do you see? In other words, we have to prove beyond reasonable doubt that Mr Hitchings' chance for survival has been materially affected by the delay in diagnosis."

Mr Crowe could be seen basking in the warmth of the phrase 'We as lawyers.'

"Now! Professor?"

Never in Professor Sleight's academic life had he heard the title, professor, conferred on someone with such disdain.

"Yes?"

"Professor, turning to the issue of causation. We have heard that there had been a delay in the diagnosis of colon cancer. We have heard that this delay is approximately 2 years. We have seen that, at diagnosis, Mr Hitchings had very advanced cancer. Tell us, if you would professor, what the stage of Mr Hitchings' cancer would have been if there had been no negligence and therefore no delay in referral by the GP."

"I believe that he would have had a locally less advanced tumour."

"Meaning, meaning, meaning professor?"

"Meaning that I think that if there had been an early diagnosis then it would have been a T2 tumour. It would have invaded through the bowel wall but not deeply. The grade would have not changed as tumours generally have the same microscopic appearance at all stages of their development."

"And would have there been any spread of the cancer if an early diagnosis had been made?"

"That's a good question and a difficult question to answer."

The barrister smirked.

'Good question. Quite so. These professor chappies, they're not the only smart cookies on the block.'

"Do proceed professor."

"I think that there would have been liver spread even if there had been an early diagnosis."

"What!" gasped Mrs Hitchings.

"Two year delay and no difference? I can't believe that you're saying that, professor. My poor Alex, he died didn't he, died, and he might not have died if that disgusting GP hadn't ignored his problem. I really can't believe that you're saying that, professor, can't believe it."

"Mr Crowe, do take Mrs Hitchings outside so that she can compose herself, would you, there's a good chap."

Mr Crowe shuffled to his feet.

But Mrs Hitchings had composed herself and wouldn't need to be taken outside, thank you very much. She glared at the professor.

"I am so sorry Mrs Hitchings. I know it seems incredible that the delay might not have made any difference to Mr Hitchings, but let me explain the logic if I may, please let me explain.

"Now I do hope that you understand that I am asked here today to give my opinion as an impartial expert witness. I am beholden to give my evidence to the Court. I have potentially, if the case proceeds, to stand up in Court, in front of the judge, and explain my conclusions and back them up with learned references. It's no good me giving an opinion that's biased and not based on fact. That opinion wouldn't stack up simply because it wasn't the truth!

"And what's worse, another pathologist could give the truth and my opinion would be drummed out of court. So I have to be objective and give my view dispassionately. That's my job."

"Professor Sleight!" the barrister boomed.

"Do, please, stick to the point. I have asked you if there is causation in this matter. Well. Is there causation?"

"I am sorry that Dr Rosenberg isn't here to help us on this. I can give an opinion as to stage but it is the oncologist who should be defining the outcome."

"Dr Sleight ..."

Professor Sleight was aware of his demotion ... and its cause.

"And furthermore, Dr Sleight, it is I who will decide when we need to consult with the oncologist.

"Dr Sleight. Can you, or can you not, tell us what the stage of the tumour would have been if there had been an early diagnosis of colon cancer?"

"As I have said ... there would have been liver spread."

"And the stage, Dr Sleight?"

"Liver spread."

Professor Sleight was puzzled as to why he had to repeat his description of the staging of Mr Hitchings' cancer and then realised that despite his explanation, in all probability, the barrister hadn't the faintest understanding of what was meant by the staging of cancer.

"I see. Why is it then, doctor, that there would have been liver spread even if there been no delay in diagnosis?"

"The reason is that colon cancer grows very slowly. It takes many years to evolve and spread. There have been studies in which patients with spread of their cancer have been followed without being treated ..."

"Without being treated?"

"Yes, it happens sometimes that people don't want to go through treatment because, for example, they do not want to have to put up with the side effects of chemotherapy or endure the rigors of surgery."

"Proceed, professor."

Professor Sleight took note of the fact of his promotion.

" ... And in this situation, doctors have measured the rate of doubling in growth of the tumour."

"How so, do say?"

"For example, if the patient who is not having treatment is kept under clinic review and has scans on a regular basis, then we can follow through time, the serial changes in the size of his tumour. We can measure by CT scan or by ultrasound, the dimensions of his tumour and by repeated CT or ultrasound, see how his tumour develops over time.

"The evidence about the rates of growth of the tumour that we find from CT scans and ultrasound is supported from laboratory evidence on the rate at which colon cancer cells multiply. We find that most of the cell lines are slowly growing.

"From all this evidence we conclude ..."

"Yes professor ... you conclude?"

"Yes, as I was saying, we conclude that colon cancer grows extremely slowly with a doubling time of about 90 days."

"And ..."

"And as colon cancer grows so slowly, it is likely, because Mr Hitchings had such extensive spread of cancer to his liver that the cancer had, as it were, already gone to the liver at the time when he first went to see his GP with rectal bleeding."

"What, professor! Surely not! I can't believe it. Two years delay and not a bloody bit of difference to what happened. Poor Alex, my poor, darling Alex and him so sick at the end ..."

"He died peacefully, I gather Mrs Hitchings?"

"You might call it that!" said Mrs Hitchings.

" ... It's true that he didn't suffer but he died, and he died because of that doctor not recognising that he had a real problem.

" ... It's too late for Alex, but can't you do something to stop him doing the same thing to anyone else?"

"Yes, Mrs Hitchings, we will, I assure you that we will." interrupted Mr Crowe.

"We'll write to his professional body and alert them to his practice standards. We'll write to the General Medical Council."

"Fat lot of good that'll do ... they're all in it together. It'll be covered up. I'll write to the papers. Something has to be done. Something has just got to be done."

"But, professor, it seems to go against sense, are you sure that an early diagnosis would not have made a difference.

"I don't think it would, but you see I am only a pathologist, and you really should ask the oncologist his views about whether the outcome would have been any different with less bulk of disease. That's not my area of expertise you know ...

"And I gather that you will be in touch with Dr Rosenberg about causation..." added Professor Sleight,

"But only if you decide that you need to be.

"After all ... it's as you said ...

"'It is I who will decide when we need to consult with the oncologist ...'"

Chapter 6
Coming Through

Jane is 55 and works in advertising. Jane is great fun, really bright, really pretty, with a gamin bob, ski jump nose and peek-a-boo eyes. She is one of those unusual people in the industry who haven't lost their job by the age of 40, an industry where you are only useful when you're young. But brains and experience are sometimes of value in advertising's zero calorie, turbo granola, biodegradable, corporate world, and Jane has survived all the culls and all the mergers to run a business with a thousand employees. She works enormously hard, drives an eco-friendly Ferrari and is divorced. She says about her marriage,

"You know, I used to stay at work until about 10 or 11 o'clock. It was so interesting, such fun. I'd come home. My husband would be there. So was dinner. He'd been home since 6:30 or 7:00. Then one day I came home and there was no Tom. There was a cold dinner. He'd left me. He'd left me because he thought that I felt that my work was more important than he was."

Jane had private healthcare insurance as part of the company benefits that came with her table at The Ivy. Mammography was part of the private healthcare benefit programme. She hadn't liked the mammography process, which squeezed and pressed at her breasts. Her doctor's receptionist had called her after the health screen and asked her to come up to clinic. That was scary. She knew that there was going to be trouble. She sat with her GP and he explained that the X-ray films had shown a little area of …

"Microcalcification in the right breast."

Jane was not amused by the idea of microcalcification. What on earth was he talking about?

The GP explained that there were little deposits of a substance like chalk within the breast tissue which caused the microcalcification, and were an indication that unfortunately … there was … a possibility of a growth.

"You mustn't worry, though,"

… which is, of course, the most worrying thing that a doctor could possibly say, and as he talked, Jane felt the twist and scream of fear trampling in great hobnail boots around her stomach.

Breast cancer is the commonest cancer of women, affecting one million women each year worldwide. In the United Kingdom there are about 45,000 women a year diagnosed with breast cancer and the life time risk of developing the disease is about 1 in 10. One way that breast cancer is diagnosed is through screening. Screening was introduced in the United Kingdom about 25 years ago as part of an election campaign initiative. The Tory government wanted to impress the female electorate that they were doing something for women's health and allegedly spent 20 times more on the advertising campaign that showed that the Tories cared for women than they spent on mammogram equipment that actually *meant* that they cared.

At the time of the campaign, most doctors thought that there was a significant downside to screening, and were against mass screening. This is because screening for breast cancer, which is by mammography, involves the use of X-rays which cause cancer, and the radiation dosage used at the time put women at a significantly increased risk of developing breast cancer from mammography itself. This increased risk was thought to outweigh any advantage of screening mammography. However, the roar and rush of the election campaign's needs overwhelmed the whispers of the doctors, and mammography was introduced.

So what happened as a result of the introduction of screening? Bizarrely the politicians were right and the doctors were wrong. The Tories 'did good', and the number of breast cases diagnosed doubled. Paradoxically this doubling led to a dramatic fall in death rates because breast cancers were detected at an earlier stage and, in breast cancer diagnosis, smaller is better in terms of survival chance. In the years since the introduction of screening, although the number of women diagnosed with breast cancer increased dramatically, the survival rate also increased equally dramatically, and death rates fell by about 30%. The current estimate is that the screening programme probably saves 1,500 women from dying of cancer each year in the United Kingdom. Screening now uses low dosages of radiation, and the risk of developing cancers from mammography is negligible.

The current recommendation is that screening is only available for women under 65 years of age. The irony is that the risk of breast cancer increases with age, although there is a minor plateauing of age risks around the time of the menopause. The arguments for not screening women over 65 are entirely economic. Older women have needs and pensions, and these needs and pensions are a burden to the State. Young women work, and this is a benefit to the State.

Although Jane had private healthcare insurance, she was a Camden Socialist who was committed to the NHS. Her GP referred her to the local hospital. She had been sent to see a surgeon under the 'Two week cancer wait' referral rule. This system had been put in place to improve outcomes for cancer patients. The surgeon was most jolly with her. He asked whether she'd felt the lump herself, and not waiting for any answer, asked her about the value of her company's shares.

Jane lay on a hard plastic couch behind flimsy floral screens and the surgeon examined her breasts. There was no apology for cold hands. Jane had always liked her breasts. They were her breasts,

'Goodness, what is he doing?'

With his right hand flattened against her breast, the surgeon inched his hand round, pressing at her breasts, the one without the microcalcification first. Then the oddest thing, thought Jane, as the surgeon changed his technique and felt her breasts with the tips of his fingers, pushing deep into her flesh. This, doctors are taught to do in order to find smaller, less obvious lumps.

"There! Got it!" said the surgeon, and then without any reassurance or comfort, said

"Now, I'm just going to put a little tiny needle into the breast dear."

The surgeon had felt a small lump at the edge of Jane's breast, out towards her armpit. He took a syringe from a plastic tray, and put a needle on the end of the syringe. It looked like an awfully big needle. He pinched Jane's breast between his fingers at the point where he'd felt the lump, and then, with a sharp movement, pierced the skin with the needle and pushed into the breast. Although it hurt a little, but hardly at all, the intrusion of the needle seemed to Jane to be such an affront, such an invasion of her self. The surgeon pulled back on the syringe, and a little spurt of blood entered its chamber. As he had pushed the needle into her breast, the surgeon had felt tissue resistance to the needle change from that of putty to grit. This characteristic change told the surgeon that Jane had cancer. He then withdrew the syringe and the attached needle.

A lady in a white coat had appeared next to the surgeon. Jane wasn't sure where she had come from. It seemed as though she'd been beamed in from Betelgeuse. The woman took the needle and syringe from the surgeon. Jane turned her head to see her squirt the contents of the syringe onto four glass slides, little dots of blood and fat, spattering from the syringe. The woman smeared these dots across each of the four slides using the edge of another slide to make a bloody trail on the glass.

"What's she doing?" asked Jane.

"I found a little lump in your breast, I'm afraid dear. What I've done is to take cells from the lump. These have been smeared and spread out onto the slides. We will look under the microscope now and see what is there. Please get dressed dear."

Jane thought that he could have explained what he was doing before he jabbed me with that bloody great needle. Still …

So Jane got dressed and sat listening to the surgeon's words. They seemed to be drifting in from another room. It all appeared to be happening to another person.

"We should have the results quite soon. There is definitely a lump, and it needs to come out. That's done under anaesthetic, and you should be in and out of hospital within a couple of days. All right? Any questions?"

Jane, of course, had no questions. She felt absolutely numbed by the process, but in some way strangely comforted by the fact that everything was automatic and would be sorted out. The surgeon, in between moments of real concern of how the FTSE 100 had fallen that morning, had made assessments about Jane's surgical needs. He had seen that the lump was small and Jane's breasts were relatively large and he told her that,

"I hope to save your breast ... with any luck, but we won't know till we're in theatre."

The surgeon nodded for emphasis on the word 'theatre'.

'How macabre', thought Jane.

'Theatre ... so it's a show, a play, a charade.'

The surgeon hoped that she would be a suitable candidate for wide local excision of the tumour. This is an operation where the tumour and a surrounding wedge of normal breast tissue are removed. He'd had a patient earlier in the morning, where the lump was large and the breast was small. For this woman, unfortunately, it would have been impossible to take out the lump without a major cosmetic defect and, for this earlier patient, more extensive surgery was required. This meant that the whole breast would have to be removed and immediate plastic surgery performed to replace the breast tissue with a flap of normal tissue swivelled round from the back to fill the gap where breast had been removed.

Jane left the clinic to find her car clamped.

"DAMMIT."

And she sat on the curb, feet in a puddle, and cried.

Meanwhile the cells taken from her breast were being looked at by a pathologist and these cells were, unfortunately, malignant. With this information, the surgeon knew that as well as removing the malignant lump, he would also have to take lymph nodes from Jane's armpit. In addition to blood the body has circulating fluid called lymph. Lymph drains from body tissues to fragile vessels called lymph channels which are interrupted at various points by lymph nodes. Lymph from the breast drains into lymph nodes in the armpit and, in the draining process, may carry malignant cells to these nodes.

A date was given for surgery. Jane made arrangements for her cleaning lady to look after her cat, packed her overnight bag, and was admitted to hospital for surgery. She was amazed at how quickly everything was organised, and this speeding up of a process that used to take many weeks, is as a result of government initiatives over the last decade.

Jane had been told to come into the hospital not having had breakfast. Patients are starved because an anaesthetic cannot be given on a full stomach. There is a risk of vomiting with anaesthesia and the possibility of inhaling stomach contents into the lung is clearly best avoided, so that's why patients fast.

Jane's tummy was rumbling as she was greeted by a pretty nurse, wearing too much makeup and rather awful green eye shadow, and shown her bed. The nurse explained that she was to undress and put on a hospital gown. The nurse measured her blood pressure and temperature, and checked that she had signed her consent for the operation.

'How strange,' she thought, 'The place doesn't smell of hospitals.'

"They'll be coming for you soon, so why not make yourself comfortable in the bed?"

With that the nurse left, and Jane surreptitiously prodded her breasts wondering what on earth the scar would be like. She had been mostly OK about things but at this moment, with the proximity of surgery looming, she was scared shitless that she'd lose her breast.

Twenty years ago it was quite routine for patients with breast cancer to lose the whole of their breast. The operation was called a mastectomy. Over the years there have been clinical trials where the survival of patients treated by radical mastectomy, which is an operation that removes the breast and all the muscles underneath the breast, have been compared to a less mutilating operation called a simple mastectomy. It was found by these trials that simple mastectomy, which is removal of the breast alone, was as effective as radical mastectomy in terms of overall patient survival. Within the different clinical trials groups, comparisons were made of the risks of local recurrence of the tumour and cancer spread. When radical mastectomy and simple mastectomy patients were contrasted, survival and local recurrence rate was found to be exactly the same. With this conclusion, the next stage of trial work was to compare the benefits of excision of the tumour alone, without removal of the breast, together with radiotherapy to the tumour cavity, to mastectomy, and the survival and local recurrence rates were again found to be the same.

This evolution of surgical techniques had taken place over a 40 year period. It had been pioneered in the 1930s by Geoffrey Keynes, John Maynard Keynes' brother who was also a noted collector of William Blake's water colours.

Jane was seen by a junior doctor, who took her history, examined her and consented her for surgery. There was nothing in his clothes that identified the person who was examining her as a doctor. He wore chinos and an open necked short sleeve shirt. He had a name badge that made him look like an employee in a chip shop. Jane wanted the reassurance of a proper doctor in a white coat. There were no white coats it seemed, and so maybe there was no reassurance. Jane wondered about that.

A nurse came in with Jane's pre-med. The pre-med contains two drugs, one to dry up lung secretions, which reduces the risk to the lung of the complications of anaesthesia, and the second drug which helps the patient to relax. The injection was given, but Jane noticed no real effects apart from a dry mouth. She certainly didn't feel relaxed. An hour later, a porter rolled a wheelchair into the ward. Jane stopped chatting with her next door bed-mate …

"Excuse me a moment,"

And went and had a pee. She clambered into her chariot, the wheelchair, and was wheeled along the corridor, in some grandeur, she felt, into the lift, and down into the operating theatre anteroom.

The anaesthetist introduced himself to her, and explained that he would be giving her a little injection which would make her fall asleep within a few seconds, and then he would intubate her.

"You are going to intubate me?"

And the anaesthetist, a smiley man with a round face and a brush over, explained …

"That means just putting a tube into your throat so that I can inflate your lungs."

For a moment, Jane had a vision of being blown up and up and up, until she floated away from the operating theatre, but she knew what the anaesthetist meant even though he was not very good at explaining himself.

The anaesthetic room was a room of brushed steel surfaces and startlingly white cupboards.

"Just a little prick."

Jane wondered about that, she'd thought him quite a nice young man, but too late, and a hollow needle was inserted into the back of her hand. White fluid was pushed into her veins.

"Just count to 10 please and you'll find yourself drifting off to sleep. We'll see you in the recovery room in no time at all."

Jane put her head back on the pillow. Her neck hurt with the tension and she wanted her mum. There she was, at the age of 55, thinking about her mum and wanting her there.

She counted, got to four, and then there was nothing.

At the beginning of Jane's nothing, the anaesthetist took a shiny instrument from his trolley, opened Jane's mouth, and inserted the instrument into her mouth so that he could have a good view of the back of her throat. He then poked a tube into her mouth which he threaded down into the back of her throat and through into her larynx.

There … she was safely anaesthetised and safely intubated.

Jane was pushed into the operating theatre, where the surgeons and scrub nurses turned in balletic synchrony to peer over face masks at the next subject for their sharp endeavours.

The surgeons checked the mammogram films confirming the size and position of the lump. Mistakes are made in surgical practice, where left legs are right legs and right kidneys left kidneys, and the surgeon really didn't want to be the one who took out the wrong mass of tissue from the wrong breast and went before the General Medical Council to explain his error. So he checked and double checked, while the Theatre Sister arranged surgical drapes over Jane's chest. Exposing Jane's breast, while thinking of exposing the nursing sister's breasts, the surgeon swabbed down Jane's breast and armpit with antiseptic, and then, through the crinkle of his rubber gloves, felt the lump in Jane's breast.

The surgeon took his scalpel and cut through the skin overlying her breast lump. The cut was made to follow the line of the breast. A point of bright blood welled from the cut, and the surgeon, spotting the bleeding point, touched an electrocautery device to the bleeding blood vessel. With an electric Splfrzzzzz, the bleeding stopped. The smell of burnt steak frizzled through the operating room. A yellow line of fat showed beneath the red line of skin. The surgeon cut deeper through fat and normal breast tissue, to expose the malignant lump, which was yellow white against the pink of normal breast tissue. The lump was excised and put into a metal kidney dish held out by the nurse. And, as Jane's chest rose and fell with the action of the ventilator, the surgeon turned and cut through the lump of cancer, bisecting it neatly with his scalpel.

The malignant lump measured about 2 cm in diameter and could be seen to nestle in and be contained by normal tissue. The surgeon was pleased that the tumour seemed completely encased by normal breast. It meant that he wouldn't have to remove more of Jane's breast. The surgeon closed the wound with neat stitches, and wiped away the blood that was staining Jane's skin. He then concentrated on her armpit and, with a neat little cut, proceeded to remove lymph nodes which look like tiny little flecks of yellow white gravel tracing along the line of the blood vessels and nerves in the armpit.

The surgeon was slightly old fashioned in his approach, removing the whole chain of nodes, which is a technique called axillary dissection. In modern surgical practice what's called a sentinel node biopsy is performed. This is where dye is injected under the skin, and tracks up into the lymph channels where it is eventually taken up by the lymph nodes. Thus outlined, the surgeon removes what's called the sentinel node, which is the marker for the pathological situation in the remaining lymph nodes. This is done to limit the side effects caused by operating on the armpit and removing the whole chain of nodes.

But surgery is over for Jane. The whole procedure had taken 35 minutes. Jane was extubated, which means that the anaesthetic tube was removed from her larynx, lifted onto a trolley and clattered into the recovery room, which is a large room where patients are sent after operations under the supervision of nurses. There, quiet and still, she recovered from her anaesthetic.

Jane woke quickly. When she awoke, her first response was to the dryness and soreness of her throat. Her second instinct was to check her breast.

She pushed down with her hand.

'Thank God', she thought.

'It's there.'

And then she felt the pain from the incision. But with the relief of knowing her breast hadn't been lopped off, she collapsed back into dreamless sleep, to wake as she was trundled in her bed through the corridors to the ward. She stayed overnight in the hospital and was told that review with her results would be next week with the surgeon.

Fate suspended, alone again, not knowing what to face, she found a taxi at the hospital entrance and went home to her cat and a concerned cleaning lady who'd made her a cake.

Being a modern sort of woman, Jane went to the Internet to find out about breast cancer, and was horrified, firstly about the amount of information that was available to her, and secondly by the fact that none of the information could be given any sort of significance or context. She was terrified by the idea of radiotherapy, scared by the concept of chemotherapy, frightened by the thought of hair loss and overwhelmed by the notion of vomiting and infection. It was so difficult to know what was right and what was wrong. A friend had told her about a patient information service called CancerBACUP run by Macmillan, and so she phoned the organisation. A very warm and sensible woman had explained to her a little about the next steps in the process of being a breast cancer patient, and promised to send her booklets that would help her understand her condition.

'Fancy,' thought Jane,

'A cancer patient! That's what I am. A cancer patient.'

The booklets did help. They were great; simple language, simple terms and a calm message of hope and sense.

The week that she had to wait until her outpatient appointment seemed unendingly long. There was bruising on the skin of her breast. Vivid purple discolouration that eased to monkey sick yellow over the week.

Then, waiting time gone, Jane sat once more in the surgeon's outpatient clinic, conscious of how alone she was in her life without the support and friendship of her husband. Her best friend was her cleaning lady. But she didn't let self pity enter into her reflection. This was how it was, and she'd deal with it, she thought.

Her name was called. She rose and went into the surgeon's consulting room.

"Lovely to see you, dear. How are you?"

And all Jane really wanted to know was that there was nothing wrong and it had all been a terrible mistake, but that wasn't to be.

"Great news for you, dear. I got that whole thing out and that should be it, really. Just a little finessing to get things finally sorted."

"And what about the armpit. Was everything all right there?" Jane found herself asking, concerned about the deception and ease of the word 'finessing'.

"Oh, yes, the armpit. Isn't it good you ask …

"One of the glands was affected but that's nothing really dear. I'm going to ask one of my friends to have a look at you and I'm sure he'll sort you out dear. Now, how's the wound? Let's have a look at it."

And as Jane lay once more on a consulting room couch, the surgeon bustled around, admiring his handiwork.

Jane dressed and sat in front of the surgeon's desk. He didn't look the sort of chap that she'd like to ask for any more information from, and she was worried that any information that might be given would be bad news.

"Yes", said the surgeon.

"All will be well. You'll see. I would like you to visit one of my colleagues because you might need a little bit more treatment dear. It's only to tidy up the edges of things. You're not to worry, dear."

That phrase, 'Not to worry, Dear', was engineered to cause the most extreme anxiety, and Jane's heart skipped and jumped, and those butterflies that seemed to be a permanent feature of life in her stomach were overwhelmed by a cyclone of catastrophic rocks that poured out of a bilious black sky.

The colleague that the surgeon wanted Jane to see was a radiotherapist. Jane's case had been discussed at a team meeting, and her future cancer treatment planned. The radiotherapist was brought into the room by the surgeon. He was brusque in his manner and very to the point. He wore horn rimmed rectangular framed glasses that slid down his purple nose and a cloak of dreadful dandruff that cascaded from his scalp onto the lapels of his blue suit. He didn't talk to Jane directly, but to the pad of notes in front of him.

"You see, dear, you'll need a little bit more treatment. Radiotherapy is given to the breast. And then after that you'll need to have some chemotherapy and perhaps some hormones. But I'm going to send you to another of my colleagues and he'll talk about that with you. OK?"

He shuffled his paper on his desk, and closed Jane's file, a sign to Jane that her time was up. She had no idea what on earth he was going on about, and thought to herself that she best just continue walking on the conveyor belt of surgery, and radiotherapy, and hopefully there would be a vista of green fields, lakes and mountains at the point where the conveyor belt hit open air. But, meanwhile, there was an awful lot of conveyor belt to shuffle along.

Why did the doctors call her dear? She had no idea, but in a strange way the term was comforting, not patronising.

Radiotherapy. The first step in the process is called planning, where the details of the treatment to be given are mapped out. Radiation dosages and distributions are calculated around the contours of Jane's breast, and also around the place where the tumour was taken away. Radiotherapy is planned so that the energy of treatment is used to treat breast tissue and spare the skin and underlying lungs and heart from radiation damage. The importance of skin sparing is that this preserves the cosmetic appearance of the breast. In past decades it was not technically possible to do this, and the skin received dosages of radiation that left it looking prematurely aged.

Jane was not sure why she had to have the radiation treatment. Nobody had told her why it was needed. She hoped that someone would explain, but no one did. So she asked one of the radiographers who were attending to her in the planning treatment room. The planning room is a little like any other medical room, with its couch and collection of medical instruments, the same except for the glowering, looming presence of a huge piece of equipment that looks like an X-ray machine. The image of Jane's breast and her overall geography are captured by this machine and fed into a planning computer, where the dosage schedule of radiotherapy treatment is fine tuned.

The radiographer helped her down from the couch.

"Hasn't anyone discussed this with you?

" ... Isn't that just typical!

" ... Doctors ...!

"The reason for the radiotherapy is to reduce the risk of the cancer coming back in your breast. Quite simple really."

"How's it given?"

"It's just like having an ordinary X-ray. You'll come up every weekday. The treatment will last moments. You'll go home and, at the end of 4 - 6 weeks, it'll all be over."

The radiographer smiled, and said

"We're done with you today. You'll get an appointment in the post with details of your treatment. See you soon."

"Well, does the treatment have any side effects?"

The radiographer smiled again.

"Do come and sit over here with me. Let's talk a little bit about the side effects. The treatment's pretty easy peasy. You won't really notice anything. Perhaps towards the end of treatment you'll have a little bit of reddening of the skin, but it shouldn't be the case. We advise you not to wash your breast with soap while treatment continues but, other than that, everything should be fine. You should be aware, though, that you might feel a bit tired as the treatment process itself is exhausting. Many people stop work during treatment, but others soldier on. Why don't you just take it a day at a time and see how you get on."

"Is there anything I should do about my diet or …?"

"No. Don't worry about anything. Just carry on normally."

'Normally!' thought Jane.

'Chance would be a fine thing!

'Normally! If only!'

So Jane went home and in due time, the appointment for radiotherapy arrived, and the morning of the first radiotherapy session dawned. The smiling receptionist directed her towards the basement of the building and Jane descended in the lift to the radiotherapy bunker. The radiographers met her as she emerged from the lift and walked with her along a winding corridor to the radiotherapy treatment room.

"Why's it so deep down?" said Jane

"It's so there's no radiation risk to anyone else. There's 30 feet of barium impregnated concrete between the radiotherapy treatment machine and the ground floor".

Jane was rather encouraged by the thought that there would be no risk to anyone else, and that 30 feet of concrete was a sufficiency for everyone else …

'But what about me?' she thought.

'What about the risk to me?'

Jane was led by a radiographer into the radiotherapy treatment room. The room was about 20 feet × 20 feet and dominated in its centre by a flat couch encompassed by the arc of a radiotherapy treatment machine. This looks exactly like an ordinary X-ray machine but there are of course differences in function. The radiotherapy treatment machine delivers a much higher dose of radiation than a normal X-ray machine. The rays used to treat patients take the form of energy emitted from a radioactive source, which is focused to treat the area where the cancer was, destroying tissue so that the risk of the cancer re-growing is reduced.

Jane was asked to lie down on the couch, and the radiographer, using red laser beams and a handheld button operated controlling device, moved the radiotherapy treatment machine out into position focused on Jane's breast.

"Now", said the radiographer. "It's time for you to lie really still."

So Jane lay really still. The radiographers marched quickly out of the room, and the radiation treatment room door closed tightly. Jane lay still on the couch and as the door closed a red warning light flashed on and off:

DANGER, DANGER, DANGER.

Jane worried about that. She'd been abandoned by everyone. And the red lights were warning her that this was dangerous.

Maybe she should be leaving too.

But before she could jump up from the couch and evacuate the room, a voice came out of the tannoy system, asking her to remain still. A few seconds later the same voice rang out again from the tannoy system,

"It's over. You can relax now"

'Relax now', thought Jane.

'I won't relax until I'm dead.'

The door to the treatment room opened and the radiographer said

"There. That wasn't bad, was it?"

Jane wasn't too sure about that. It seemed pretty bad to her, but at least it was over. She hadn't felt a thing but the process was just too freaky for words. Why had she got the damned thing? It wasn't fair. It just wasn't fair at all.

"So, we'll be seeing you tomorrow. Same time", said the radiographer.

"You mean there are more of these?"

"Yes. About 20 sessions in all."

So, day on day went by, and at the end of four weeks Jane had completed radiation therapy. It hadn't been too bad at all. There had been no sickness or vomiting. The explanations of what was to happen had not been the greatest. When doctors explain medical procedures to patients, communication from the medical teams is generally not the easiest for patients to understand. Doctors forget how complex and distant our language is from every day conversation. The words that we think are understandable and simple are many miles away from most people's conversational English.

The best explanations had often come from non-medical staff. The explanations can come from anyone. Often it's the porter wheeling patients to radiotherapy who might explain that, 'Actually', there would be no electrical shocks from the equipment, that reassures the patient who's been dazed and confused by the technical terms. It is amazing how this simple reassurance can be so helpful. The explanations of ward clerks and phlebotomists about the details of chemotherapy or radiotherapy, or the words of other patients who have been through a similar process, are without doubt by far the best forms of communication.

But radiotherapy was over, and now it was time for Jane to shuffle along another couple of clinic doors for conversations with a medical oncologist. Jane sat in the consulting room in the Cancer Centre talking with the medical oncologist. The Cancer Centre was unlike most people's idea of what a hospital should be. In the planning of the building, attempts had been made to make the environment patient-friendly. The formal furniture in the waiting areas was modern, and arranged around coffee tables.

The waiting room looked like the lounge in a smart club, and was in contrast to the reception areas in many medical buildings, that generally feature a collection of furniture obtained from a scrap yard, arranged around the perimeter of the room. There were comfortable leather sofas grouped together in the bright light of a triple height atrium. The waiting area smelt of coffee and cakes. The paintings on the wall were interesting. They were paintings rather than prints and hadn't been bought from Paperchase. There were potted plants and cut flowers.

It had taken some time and some thought to establish an environment that was comfortable and relaxing. There was a coffee bar that was a little like the coffee bar that you might see in a smart café in airports. The receptionists were told that their job is the most important job in the unit because it was where the patients first encountered the oncology process. They understand how it is so important to welcome the patients and make them feel comfortable.

Jane liked the place. It seemed a lot better to her than the metallic surfaces of surgery, and the cold shock of radiation therapy. She liked the medical oncologist who she noticed talked with her, without the separation of a desk.

Before the meeting with Jane the medical oncologist had taken care to carefully read through all of her medical notes and, in particular, had concentrated on the specifics of the pathology report.

The pathology report tells the doctor almost everything that he needs to know about the patient's future. The report describes the tumour grade, which details the microscopic aggressiveness of the tumour, and the tumour stage, which records its size and spread to lymph nodes. The report told the oncologist what Jane would face in her future.

The pathologist had looked down the microscope and concluded that the tumour grade as 'poorly differentiated.' This meant that all the cells looked bizarre, and were not forming the conventional structures that would normally be seen in breast tissue. The pathologist had commented about the staining of the tumour for specific receptors. These receptors, which are proteins presented on the cell's surface and in the cell's interior function by combining with other proteins and steroids and this binding process activates the cancer cell. The receptors, are for hormones such as oestrogen and progesterone, and also for a protein made by a gene mutated in cancer called an 'oncogene'. Jane's oestrogen and progesterone receptor status were negative, while the oncogene receptor staining was positive. This immediately told the oncologist that hormonal therapy would not be of any use. It would have no effect in Jane's case. The oncogene receptor protein was positive and that implied a poor prognosis.

'Poor prognosis' …

Doctor speak for …

'She's not got much of a chance'.

The tumour had spread to Jane's lymph nodes. This, together with Jane's receptor status marked out a poor future for her and underlined the importance of her having additional chemotherapy. The surgery and radiotherapy were not sufficient to give her the best chance of survival, and she needed to have everything that she could possibly have to help her.

The medical oncologist looked at Jane and saw a healthy woman who looked fit and well. The trouble with breast cancer is that you can never tell. All the normal markers that tell the doctor of a patient's fate aren't present on the face of woman with breast cancer until her illness has progressed.

'Progressed'.

That's another word whose meaning has been subverted by doctors. Progressed doesn't mean things have got better. It means that the patient's condition has worsened and is far more serious than it was.

The pathology report also gives doctors information that details prognosis. Oncologists can act on this information from the pathologist and work out their patient's prognosis by going to a website that defines survival. At this Internet site the doctor types in all of the features of a woman's breast cancer, presses a button and comes out with a precise survival chance. The figures are obtained from statistics garnered from the fate of many thousands of women. The oncologist had typed in Jane's details and found that she had a 65% chance of surviving for 10 years. This was not good news. Not good news at all at 55. He wondered if she'd ask about her chances of survival.

The oncologist liked Jane immediately. He was fond of all of his patients, but he liked her more than most. He thought about that fondness for a moment and realised that it was based on the realisation that in normal circumstances Jane was the sort of person that if he had not been married, he would have liked to have been 'friendly with' and recognising this the doctor felt disconcerted, shocked.

'Doctors have to be careful about that.' the consultant thought.

'Can't let people get too close.'

He remembered his father, who was also a doctor, talking about just this sort of thing and his father's words on the subject were just right.

'To be a good doctor, you have to feel for your patients … But not feel too much.'

'What a great summary, good old Dad!

'But … best get back to the job in hand!'

The medical oncologist smiled at Jane and asked,

"So, do you know why you're here?".

From the look on her face it was quite clear that she had absolutely no understanding of what faced her.

"Look doc, I know nothing. I'm just going with the flow. I don't want to know about the future. I am going a day at a time.

"But one thing that you can help me with please … Why have I got this bloody thing?"

So what are the causes of breast cancer? These have been clearly known for many years. The first associations were made in the mediaeval period when nuns were noted to get breast cancer. This observation defines one of the major risk factors for the development of breast cancer, which is not having children. The reason for this is that a significant proportion of breast cancer is dependent upon a woman's "hormonal environment". The gross hormonal changes associated with pregnancy are protective against the development of breast cancer. Strangely, this beneficial effect ceases if a first child is born to a mother over 30 years of age. In the future, the incidence of getting breast cancer will clearly increase because there is currently so much pressure upon women to contribute to household economies and compete with men in the workplace, so that the age of first pregnancy is getting later and later.

Diet is also very strongly associated with the risk of breast cancer. The chance of developing breast cancer is reduced by about a factor of two in women who are vegetarian. Obesity is also strongly linked with breast cancer, and women who are more than twice the normal weight for their height and size are twice as likely to get breast cancer than a woman of average weight.

There is a strong genetic basis to the development of breast cancer. Women who have more than two affected first degree relatives, that is a mother, sister or aunt, with breast cancer, are also twice as likely to develop breast cancer as women without affected family members. There are about four major groups of genes that cause breast cancer and the genes about which most are known are called BRCA1 and 2. Mutations in these genes occur in about 5% of all breast cancer cases, and for women with mutation in these genes, the risk of developing breast cancer, and incidentally the risk of getting ovarian cancer, exceed 80%.

There is considerable good news, for breast cancer patients, and this is that overall, over the last 20 years, the chance of a woman surviving breast cancer has increased significantly. Survival chance has risen from about 65% to well over 80%, and this bottom line is frequently lost in the awful fear that quite understandably echoes from a diagnosis of breast cancer.

"So you want to know why you're here. Seems like a reasonable question!"

And the doctor smiled. Jane warmed to him; she liked the doctor best of all the clinicians that she'd seen, she liked his crooked smile and delicate hands. She found herself thinking …

The doctor described to Jane the additional treatment that she would need.

"How do you know that that's the right treatment for me?"

"That's a very good question."

Over the last 30 years doctors have investigated the benefits of chemotherapy given to patients with breast cancer around the time of their diagnosis. These are called adjuvant treatments. Investigations have proceeded in an evolutionary way and successful treatments selected. Groups of women have been randomised to receive different drug regimens and, slowly, the best hormonal and chemotherapy treatments have evolved and been selected.

Treatments have changed with the discovery of new drugs for the treatment of breast cancer, and it is estimated that the addition of chemotherapy, particularly to a woman with spread of her disease to lymph nodes, gives a benefit of perhaps 4 to 7% in terms of their survival chance. This means that an additional four to seven woman in every hundred treated will survive as a result of receiving chemotherapy compared with what would happen without chemotherapy treatment. Current chemotherapy treatment involves the use of multiple drugs, given every three to four weeks, for a period of four to six months.

The doctor explained to Jane the treatment regimen that would be used and its side effects, which included nausea and vomiting, hair loss and infection. Nausea and vomiting is a physiological response to a dose of poison … which is how the body perceives chemotherapy drugs. It's an attempt by the body to get rid of noxious substances. Drugs have been developed to control nausea and vomiting, and nowadays, even with the worst sort of treatment programme, just 10 to 20% patients suffer from this side effect.

Hair loss is unfortunately inevitable for many of the treatment programmes. It usually comes three to four weeks after the start of chemotherapy, and is most dispiriting. Women are strongly advised to get a wig and practise wearing it before they lose their hair, so when hair loss comes they are accustomed to the use of the wig. Hair will always re-grow and two to three months after the completion of chemotherapy, the glimmer of a crew cut appears on the scalp.

One of the most important of the other side effects of chemotherapy is infection. This comes because chemotherapy has an effect upon the bone marrow. It suppresses the formation of all of the blood forming cells. The most important of these are the white cells, which fight infection. Without white cells, patients are more susceptible to infection as a result of cancer treatment. Infection manifests by the patient feeling as if they have the most awful flu. If it's recognised and treated, then there is virtually no risk to the patient. If it's left then the risk of overwhelming infection are enormous and the patient could die. Treatment takes the form of admission to hospital and the use of antibiotics.

The doctor explained all this to Jane, and then took her down to show her the treatment area in the Oncology Centre. Patients were treated in seats that looked a little bit like an airline seat. Inbuilt into the seat were charging points for iPods and laptops. Video screens were available to view DVDs.

The place looked good to the consultant, he was proud of it; that was where he worked.

However, for Jane, it was a heart stop moment as she gazed at the chairs and the patients, with their intravenous lines attached to clear plastic delivery sets linked to bags of chemotherapy on drip stands, and saw her fate.

"This is what we have at the moment, Jane. This is how treatment is. In the future, it won't be like this. There are so many things that we have now for our patients, but didn't previously. There's hope, Jane, I promise."

The consultant could see that Jane was shocked. Her eyes were lowered to the ground and she was quiet.

"But why can't I have hormone treatment instead?" she asked.

Hormone treatment has also undergone some refinement over the last 30 years. It used to be commonplace for patients to receive additional hormonal treatment with a drug called tamoxifen. Tamoxifen works by partly blocking the binding of circulating female hormones to their cellular receptors. In normal circumstances this binding process would lead to the division of cells, and this reproductive process is not exactly what's wanted in cancer patients! Rather, it's the opposite: we want the cancer cells to die! Tamoxifen blocks the process of cancer cell growth and multiplication. In recent times, another series of drugs have been developed that add to the effects of tamoxifen. They are called aromatase inhibitors, and these act by blocking the chemical steps that lead to the production of the hormones. The best of benefits from hormonal therapy is from combining tamoxifen and aromatase inhibitor treatments. This benefit, just like the benefit of chemotherapy, has been shown by large scale clinical trials. The consultant explained to Jane that these were not treatments that were suitable for her, in view of the unique characteristics of her tumour, which was hormone receptor negative. Hormone treatment won't work in hormone receptor negative patients.

"However", he said,

"There is something that will help that comes from modern times."

Jane would need additional treatment, with herceptin. Herceptin was developed in the last 20 years by a group of medical scientists who identified the presence of a growth factor receptor on the surface of breast cancer cells. This receptor, when activated, drives breast cancer growth. The scientists went on to develop and prove the efficacy of treatment, such as herceptin, directed against this receptor. Jane would need this treatment in order to get the best of benefits from adjuvant treatment. The consultant explained to her that this also would have side effects additional to the chemotherapy, and the most important were those on the heart. For this reason, she would need monitoring of her heart during the process of chemotherapy. Additional scans would be needed,

"But Jane, you are not to worry. We now know that these cardiac changes, if they come are reversible."

"Thanks doc. I am really glad they are reversible. Great news!

" ... What a business!" she sobbed.

"Seems like there's no end to it all."

"There is an end ..." the consultant said.

" ... There will be an end ...

" ... It will be over ...

" ... You will come through ... You *will* come through."

Chapter 7
Here's Henry

They're in the consulting room, it's where everything happens … and there's Henry, sitting on the edge of his chair, fists clenched, glowering, furious, enraged.

Henry is 62 years old. Henry knows he's a success, knows he's a success in everything that he does. Henry is always in the driving seat, in control, running things. The driving seat is mostly in a Bentley. The driving is from the office to the restaurant and also from the restaurant to the office. That's Henry's favourite exercise: driving to restaurants.

Henry didn't look like the sort of person that was home much. He was wearing a beautiful blue suit, quite the best thing to have ever come out of Savile Row, a Hermes tie, and Italian loafers. There was Tiffany gold at his wrists. His face glistened with moisturiser. He was glossy with an affluence that resonated from him in diamant´ waves around the waiting room. And then there was the aftershave. Henry is definitely bold font and capitalised.

A moment before, the doctor had come out of the consulting room to say …

"Hello", and asked Harry in to his room.

Henry was with his wife. The invitation was for her too of course.

Henry looked up from the pink pages of the *Financial Times*, and said to her,

"You wait here. I'll see him alone."

J. Waxman, *The Elephant in the Room*,
DOI 10.1007/978-0-85729-895-9_7,
© Springer-Verlag London Limited 2012

He shook the doctor's hand and the grip was firm. Too firm. The strength of his grip told the doctor of Henry's anxiety.

Henry led the way into the consulting room. He banged the door open and as the doctor followed him through the doorway, the door swung into his face. There were no apologies from Henry. He stomped to the consulting desk, pulled out a chair, glowered, crossed his legs and ran his hands through the puffs of dyed hair that billowed from the sides of his skull to nestle, sculpted and draped across the prairie plains of his baldness.

"I just don't believe it," he growled.

"I am not going through that. What's the point?"

Henry thumped the desk with a clenched fist.

Henry … he was so upfront. It was all there, without pretence, without affectation. He didn't care what anyone thought about him. He was just Henry, and he was going to be Henry, so the rest of you could take it or leave it.

The doctor had flicked through his records before seeing him. It was always best to be briefed. Doctors don't like surprises. It makes them look foolish, fallible, flaky and ultimately unbelievable.

He'd read that Henry had undergone a recent annual medical. It is common for successful business people to have annual medical checks. These checks were particularly pleasing to most business people because they didn't have to pay for it, the business did.

Screening medicals are not frequently carried out in the general male population. There are many reasons for this. Firstly, there is the apathy of men to deal with. Men are generally unconcerned about pre-emptively sorting out health problems. So much so, that it's thought that just 2 to 5% of the UK male population have screening assessments carried out. Secondly, men are relatively justified in their apathy because academic studies have shown that the value of screening is contentious. The only proven gain, apart from the money that flows into the coffers of the practices that offer screening tests, is in the detection of high blood pressure and the identification of ear wax. These two conditions, if treated, lead to health benefits ... a reduction in cardiovascular causes of death and cures for deafness. Some men would argue that the treatment of deafness is not helpful in the context of domestic life where they would prefer to remain unable to hear the voices of their partners and continue in the potting shed with the short wave radio on.

Henry's annual medical tests had produced an abnormal finding. He had had a battery of blood tests. One of the tests had been for prostate cancer and this had come up with a result that was high. This had led to his referral for an opinion and then another opinion and then a third opinion. Henry hadn't liked anything that had been said to him by the doctors.

The test is for PSA. PSA is a chemical that is made by the prostate. The prostate's normal role is to make a fluid, rich in sugars, which nourishes sperm on their exciting journey into the wild, wild, world. PSA is secreted into the prostatic fluid. Semen clots, without the presence of PSA, which has the necessary biological function of keeping the semen fluid. If semen were to clot then all the delicate, microscopic tubes that carry it would clog up. So in many ways PSA could be considered to be like Harpic for the 'male bits'.

The normal range for PSA in blood is up to 4ng/ml. The normal range increases with age. It is not government policy for men to be screened for prostate cancer. Government policy is right for many reasons and this is because the blood test that's used to screen is inaccurate. The testing of normal populations has to have a decent level of accuracy. So, if you were to look ... and the only way to look is by carrying out a biopsy ... at the prostates of people with a PSA result in the range 4 to 10, then just 25% would have a cancer. In the range 10 to 40, just 40% of people would have cancer. So, the result is a lot of anxiety and discomfort, without a major chance of a cancer diagnosis. This summation of anxiety and discomfort is compounded by a body of considerable counter intuitive evidence that the early detection of prostate cancer and its subsequent treatment, probably does not lead to a significant increase in overall life expectancy.

The doctor continued reading. The GP's letter told him that Henry had a test result of 8ng/ml. He'd been to see a surgeon who had told him that he needed a biopsy of the prostate and would be likely to require surgery. Henry didn't like that idea and had gone to see another surgeon who had told him the same thing.

The GP had asked for a third opinion, which was the current consultation.

So that was the background. So now let's go to the foreground. Here's Henry. He is the entire foreground.

Henry was fuming.

"My appointment was for 10.30. It's now *10.35*."

He stared ostentatiously at the most enormous gold Rolex that had ever been made and snarled.

"I apologise." said the doctor,

Henry seemed to relax. Dr Jones had been late because on the way to delivering the kids to school he had realised that he'd forgotten his son's football kit and with a hand brake turn, he'd had to make a diversion back home to avoid disasters. But Dr Jones was not very late!

"Well, you've read my notes. What do you think?"

Henry drummed his fingers on the edge of the desk.

"What do you think?" countered the doctor.

"I know what you are going to say. But before you start going on ... the reason she's out there is because she doesn't know that I have been on Viagra for 12 years."

"She doesn't know?"

"No reason to tell her is there? I know about surgery so before we go any deeper into things, just remember she doesn't know, OK?"

"Got it!

"Would you like me to ask her in now?

"YES!"

"What should I tell her is the reason for her being outside?"

"No need to tell her anything. She knows I had to talk about a private matter."

Sounded like a great relationship. But it was understandable that he couldn't admit to impotence. This involvement with his hidden secret made the doctor's life difficult. He wasn't starting out honestly; he was colluding with Henry's story and becoming part of his plot. Put everything on a tricky base before starting out.

Henry and Stella.

She is about 60, lots of makeup, Chanel jacket, a short fur coat and tall court shoes with golden heels. A cigarette smoker's voice. No doubt in a few years' time the doctor would be seeing her too.

They go through Henry's story. The doctor asks him about his urinary system, how well and how often he pees, whether he wakes at night to urinate, and whether he has trouble starting or stopping peeing. This tells the doctor whether or not Henry has symptoms from changes to his prostate. The prostate sits at the bottom of the bladder. The bladder can be imagined as a football attached to a long connecting tube threading through the prostate and then into the penis. Entry into this tube, which is called the urethra, is made difficult by any enlargement of the prostate. This can then lead to a slow urinary stream and frequency because of difficulty in emptying the bladder completely. Entry into the urethra is controlled by two sets of valves. When a prostate cancer is present, the urethral valves can become infiltrated by cancer and stiffen. This leads to trouble stopping and starting peeing.

Henry had no trouble at all. He slept through the night except apparently when Stella woke him because his snoring was getting too much to bear.

The doctor asks about Henry's sex life. He does so because prostate cancer can cause impotence. Although he knows Henry's answer to this question, he still asks it because it's important to register with Stella that the treatment of prostate cancer can affect sexual function. This may be due to extension of the tumour of the prostate to neighbouring nerves and blood vessels which are involved in the mechanics of the production of an erection. Henry has had difficulty with his sex life for many years and the length of time during which he had had trouble suggested another cause for impotence other than prostate cancer.

"Works like clockwork. No problem at all."

"I'll say." said Stella.

"Wish someone would throw away the key."

"The key?" Asked the doctor.

" … To the clockwork."

Henry was then asked whether he had any other medical problems. He had slightly raised blood sugars that required tablets to control, and then was asked about his family … asked what his mother and father had died from and whether or not there was cancer in the family.

His mother had died from breast cancer and his father from a stroke. There was no prostate cancer in the family. If Henry's father had died from prostate cancer then his risk of getting prostate cancer would be increased by a third and would more than double if he had a brother with prostate cancer.

So by talking to Henry the doctor had found out quite a lot. He had no symptoms and no family history so with any luck the odds were in his favour that he didn't have a cancer.

"Would you like me to examine you?"

"If you must."

"I don't have to but it does help me come to a view."

"You guys, there must be something wrong with you lot. You are all fixated on bottoms."

So Henry lay on his side on the examination couch, and curled up in a ball, knees drawn high up into his chest.

"It would help if you lowered your pants." said the doctor,

"Kinda tricky with the trousers on."

A small smile cracked the anger.

Gloves on, always a good thing, jelly on the index finger tip, the doctor pushed his finger into Henry's bottom.

When the doctor was a medical student he had watched a senior clinician harangue a junior doctor on a ward round for not carrying out a rectal examination on a patient. The accompanying retinue of juniors, nurses and students held their collective breath in their embarrassment.

"Sister" said the senior.

"Glove."

While continuing to berate the junior doctor, head turned towards that unfortunate doctor, and paying no attention to the course of his examining finger, he carried out an exemplary rectal assessment …

But this was an assessment that was not quite textbook. With his finger's march he had managed to insert his tie into the patient's bottom. The simple error was noticed at the point when the consultant had been dragged a couple of inches towards the patient by an unseen and silky force.

"Sister." he said.

"Scissors."

And he continued on the ward round with a shortened tie. This sort of thing would not happen nowadays. A lot of bizarre and bonkers things happened in those days.

About an inch in, the doctor's finger came across the contour of Henry's prostate. In normal men of Henry's age, normal men without prostate cancer, the prostate has a smooth surface. The shape and size is that of a small apricot, with a deep grove running from top to bottom. Henry's prostate was the size of a large apricot and it had two little bumps on its surface. These bumps shouldn't have been there, shouldn't have been there at all.

"Well?" asked Henry.

The doctor's finger hadn't left the confines of Henry's bottom.

"Why don't we talk about things when you are dressed?"

So Henry got dressed and returned to his chair.

"Well?"

"I think you should have a biopsy."

"Why? Do you think that there's a problem?"

There was no way of avoiding Henry's question but the doctor had a go!

"What have you been advised by the other doctors?"

"They all said the same thing."

"You know it's unusual for three doctors to have the same opinion."

"Hmm. Tell me then …"

So the doctor explained that the PSA test result was raised and that the prostate didn't feel as it should do in a normal man. But before the doctor could get very much further, Henry interrupted with ...

"So what's it like, the biopsy?"

A biopsy of the prostate is carried out under ultrasound imaging guidance. The same sort of equipment that is used to take pictures of babies in the womb is used to image the prostate. The imaging probe is inserted a short distance into the anus and injections of local anaesthetic are given into the prostate. This is a little uncomfortable but for some the indignity of the procedure far exceeds the minor feeling of pressure that accompanies the injection. Without the anaesthetic the procedure is pretty painful. Then, with the help of the ultrasound images which can be compared to SatNav for the prostate, thin, hollow needles are inserted into the prostate and cores of tissue removed with the needles.

These cores are examined under the microscope and, according to their appearance, so a diagnosis is made. Cancer looks like normal tissue but is subtly different, different in terms of the lack of organisation of the cells which do not form nice neat glands, and also in the look of the individual cells which appear to be dividing more actively than they should be doing. The appearance of the cells is graded and issued with a number by the pathologist assessing them. The grading is called the Gleason score which ranges from 1 to 5. The higher the number the less like normal tissue the biopsy material is. High scores are associated with poor outcomes and low scores with better outcomes. The two most prevelant patterns of Gleason score within the prostate are used to provide a combined score.

There are risks attached to the biopsy. Infections may result. This is because the biopsy needles have to pass through the gut wall and so can carry into the prostate all the noxious bugs that you can live happily with when they are in the gut but not when they have been embedded into the prostate. The patient with this sort of problem feels like he has terrible flu a few hours after the biopsy. He then needs to be treated with intravenous antibiotics in hospital; if he doesn't get treated then he can die. The biopsy can also cause bleeding which usually settles quickly. In some patients this can be very severe and require a blood transfusion to correct. The bleeding is generally minor and patients may notice blood appearing in their urine or semen. These risks of bleeding and infection are about 1 to 5% ... so they are significant.

"So what happens if I don't have the biopsy?"

The doctor explained that would be Henry's choice and he would support his decision.

"Where have you gone to find out about your condition?"

"CONDITION?"

Henry expressed indignation that he should be considered to have a condition. He had spoken with one or two friends and wasn't impressed. He wasn't impressed with anything.

"Try the Prostate Cancer Charity. They have a great web site and a wonderful helpline."

More Hmm's.

And then ...

"Isn't it best to know what you are dealing with? If this was a business situation, would you be putting in £1million without knowing what you were investing in?"

"I don't deal with pocket money."

"OK ... how about £50 million."

"More like it. I'll have one of those things then."

By not naming the 'thing', Henry was dismissing the importance of the procedure, and minimising the significance of the fact of cancer itself.

So Henry went through the biopsy and came back to discuss the result. There had been no complications from the procedure and all had gone smoothly.

Henry tapped his fingers on the edge of the doctor's desk.

"Well? So what you going to tell me?"

There were to be no gentle introductions, no slow easing in, and no preliminary preamble here. Just straight in, is what the man wants ...

"I'm sorry to have to tell you that we found that there was a little cancer in the specimens."

"A little cancer!

"Sounds big to me.

"Cancer's big, doctor, it's always big, to the patient!"

That seemed to the doctor to be a reasonable, and considered summary ... but there were details that might give Henry some reason to think that hopefully, his cancer could be sorted out.

So it was explained that the biopsies had shown that he had a combined Gleason score 3 + 3 tumour occupying 20% of two of the eight cores of tissue taken from his prostate. This meant that the tumour was expected to behave in a relatively indolent manner, which is doctor speak for being mild mannered and unlikely to do the patient in, because the lower the Gleason grade the more benign the tumour.

It was also explained that Henry needed some further tests to make sure that the cancer hadn't spread. He was told that the chances of spread were low. The tests were a CT scan to assess whether there was spread to the lymph glands that drain the prostate, the motorway along which cancer cells can spread, an MR scan, which is used to define the shape of the prostate and provides images of the tumour and its extent of spread out of the prostate and a bone scan to see whether or not there was spread to bones.

The scans were carried out within a few days and as expected were negative ... in other words there were no glands that were enlarged and no bone spread. The prostate tumour looked small and hadn't breached the confines of the prostate.

"The scan results are fine."

"Is that it? How do we know they are fine?"

"That's a very good question. You see the scans just give us pictures of the shapes and sizes of internal organs. Your organs are all normal."

"Good to know something's normal!" Stella interjected.

The doctor continued.

"They don't give a microscopic image of what's going on inside the body. And it's the microscope that makes the diagnosis of cancer; it's what the cells look like, as seen under the microscopic that defines the presence or absence of cancer.

"So we know in many cancers that if glands are enlarged, they don't necessarily contain cancer cells. There is a chance of about 40% that there are no tumour cells inside those glands. And what is more perverse … we also know that if the glands are within the normal size limit, then there is the same sort of chance that the glands contain tumour, depending on the PSA level and the Gleason grade."

"How do you know?" Henry glowered.

We know from tables that give us the statistical chance of gland involvement and extension of the tumour outside of the prostate."

Henry growled at the idea of tables, statistics and chances.

"OK. What are we going to do about this then?"

"It does depend on you and your view. I can't tell you what to do."

"Look I am business man and I know about risk … tell me."

Henry crossed his legs and the doctor noticed that Henry was wearing blue suede boots. The doctor hadn't seen blue suede boots since 1978 and that was at a very dodgy party.

"I'll try and explain. The scans results are good and the PSA level and Gleason grade are in your favour. They would lead us to conclude that local treatment is possible. By local treatments we mean that you could be treated with either radiotherapy or surgery."

"What about surveillance? I have read about that. Why aren't you telling me about surveillance?"

The doctor would have told him about surveillance if he had been given just a little more time to explain things but Henry wasn't used to allowing people a little more time.

Now the difficulty is that in the situation that Henry was in, there is no evidence that early treatment prolongs survival. All the studies had shown that for a patient with the sort of tumour that Henry had, early treatment was not necessarily curative. In other words, the tumour would behave as it jolly well liked regardless of any treatment given. It could spread at a later date or remain cured even if it had been removed surgically or wiped out by radiotherapy. This is counter intuitive. You would think that treatment should be curative. The reasons for this are not known. But it is possible that the tumour cells may spread early to tissues outside of the prostate, doing so in microscopic form that cannot be detected by conventional scans, which can only identify changes in the size of internal organs by about 1 cm.

"So surveillance, which means close monitoring and starting treatment if the PSA begins to increase significantly, is a reasonable approach and it's something that commonly carried out in men older than you."

The doctor didn't add that …

'Younger men generally opt for active treatment'.

The evidence that surveillance is as good as active and early treatment is pretty sketchy. Doctors know that there is a very small advantage to surgery for those men with high Gleason grade tumours. The men with these tumours tend to do a little better with surgery but the advantage in terms of increased chance of survival is very small … just a few single figure percentage points.

The doctor watched Henry's face for signs that would tell him whether he preferred the idea of surveillance or active treatment but not a line broke on his poker face. There wasn't a clue to be had.

"So what would you do then?"

"Difficult question Henry. We try to give advice that would be the advice that we would give to our family members and give advice that we would follow ourselves."

But it's a strange thing. When doctors are polled about whether or not they would have treatment for cancer, many of them say…

'No! Thanks … but … no'.

However this is not what they tell their patients to do. They suggest that there are treatments available. But these polls have not been carried out on doctors who have cancer. With a cancer diagnosis everything changes, and when doctors are confronted by mortal illness they will, just like any human being, opt for almost anything that gives them a chance for life.

The doctor explained that he could tell Henry what he thought … and could say what he thought would be best for him but would prefer that he himself should consider the options and try to come to his own view.

"That's bloody helpful … why won't you tell me what you think?"

"In this particular situation, there is no absolute right or wrong way of going about things. There are options and you, the patient, have to make up your mind about what you really want."

"OK. I better go off and see a few more of you quacks then."

So Henry went awf and saw a radiotherapist who explained to him that he would need hormone treatment for a few months and then could be treated with radiotherapy. The radiotherapy could either be given by the use of conventional external radiation or could be given by brachytherapy. Brachytherapy is a technique where radioactive seeds are implanted in the prostate under general anaesthetic. It usually requires supplementation by external radiotherapy. The process of external radiotherapy, Henry understood, usually took six weeks to complete. People are attracted to brachytherapy because it seems so up to date, so technologically advanced. It is advanced but it's also been around for a long time, hasn't been proven to be more effective than standard external beam radiotherapy, and has the same and additional complications to standard radiotherapy.

Henry saw a surgeon who was

'Very confident he could cure me.'

Henry said that the surgeon was certain that he could get the whole thing out with no trouble at all and would use a robot to help him with the operation. The surgeon spent 10 minutes with Henry. Henry liked him. It was the businessman in the surgeon that Henry responded to. Henry explained to me that the robot allowed the surgeon to operate remotely just in the way that a kid would use a PlayStation or Xbox. The robot gave the surgeon a magnified view of the operation and reduced blood loss. The robot tied the surgeon's knots and sliced up the patient for him … to use Henry's own words. The surgeon ushered Henry away to see a nurse, a physical therapist, and a psychologist, all of whom explained in more detail how the surgeon would operate. They told Henry that there might be side effects from the surgery and that it was important to be fit before the operation took place.

Surgery causes impotence in 25% to 70% of men. It can be treated in some men. Treatment starts with drugs like Viagra, moves on to using tiny pessaries that are placed in the end of the penis, continues with injections into the penis, moves on to vacuum devices and may finish with surgically inserted inflatable rods. Radiotherapy causes impotence too, but unlike surgery this comes on gradually over many years.

The impotence caused by surgery and radiotherapy has to be dealt with as soon as possible. The longer that it's left untreated the less likely it is to respond to treatment.

Surgery can cause significant incontinence in 1 to 25% of men and this is treated by pelvic floor exercises that are similar to those that a woman practises after childbirth, and sometimes by drugs or even further operations.

"Well!" said Henry,

"What a bloody business. I tell you if I …"

And a series of stuttering expletives followed which Henry really could not be blamed for.

"I am not bloody letting that fellow near me with that blasted robot. He's not cutting me with his bloody contraption, that stupid bloody machine."

"What about the radiotherapy Henry?"

Henry had turned away to glare at his wife. He swung around to fix the doctor with venous, bulging, blue eyes.

"All right. I will have that. But none of those bloody hormones. Got it?"

The doctor got the picture. It was in many ways reasonable to do without the hormones. It had been shown that if a patient took hormonal therapy for at least two years in addition to radiotherapy then there was a survival benefit. This benefit was small and only for the nastiest grade of tumour. Henry's tumour was not of the nastiest grade. Most studies had shown that if hormone treatment was continued for two years or more then the risk of the cancer coming back in the prostate was slightly reduced for all grades of prostate cancer.

So, as the disadvantages of hormonal therapy were considerable and include impotence and loss of drive, and the advantages slight, Henry had made an absolutely balanced decision.

Henry, done his due diligence, looked at the alternatives and made his decision, had made his choice. It was the one for him. It was what he felt was the best for him as a person.

Henry had chosen radiotherapy and found himself taken up in a process that was highly technological. He didn't want brachytherapy,

"Can't see the point." he said,

"Same sort of results as bog standard treatment, but it's more complex than standard treatment to give and it seems that there are more complications."

Henry told his doctor that he had been comforted by the way that he was dealt with by the personnel that ran the scanning equipment that had probed and pried, taking up the secrets of his interior life and capturing them in digital printouts.

"Professional and considerate, courteous and kind".

Henry explained that for the first time in his adult life he felt that someone actually cared for him. The radiographers and nurses were, apparently,

'Sweet'.

"What about me Henry? Am I sweet?" asked the doctor.

"You don't care. You don't really care at all do you? You are just doing a job. They are different. They are actually helping me."

Seemed like a rather unfair point. The doctor might just have put things differently.

Henry had had a planning CT scan. It's like an ordinary CT scan with subtle differences. The patient lies on a couch and the scanner takes pictures of the area which is to be treated. The scanning process lasts about 20 minutes. The CT scanner captures the details of Henry's innards, the lines and margins, contours and cavities, in order to calculate the distribution of the radiation that he is to receive, allowing physicists to plan the treatment of his tumour. The aim is to maximise treatment to the prostate and minimise any radiation dose to the normal surrounding tissue.

The planning computer establishes what looks like an ordnance survey map, a cross section of Henry's pelvis traversed by lines demarcating radiation dosages given to specific areas of his prostate and surrounding normal tissues. The trick is to get these lines just right. You see the prostate is in very close proximity to the neck of the bladder and the lower rectum. If too much radiation is scattered to the bladder or rectum then there can be consequences. These consequences of radiation overdose include bloody diarrhoea and urinary frequency.

There is a human element to this planning process: it is not all post, post graduate, high level physics and incredible computer programs. In his planning treatment sessions, the radiotherapist will scour the treatment dose map and adjust the plan worked out by physicists using the planning software and the information obtained from the planning scan. This is the subjective part of the process. Generally radiotherapists get better results as they age ... getting used to the intricacies of the delivery of treatment, crafting the energy waves around what they see in the scans. It's as if there is an intuitive element to the planning, the skilled radiotherapist seeing the confines of the tumour in a way that is impossible to define.

The doctor remembered discussing with Julian Bloom, a most esteemed radiotherapist, why it was, that he got such good results and he said with some modesty,

"Well, I just got a little bit better."

And he did get better. He was, in his area of specialisation, the best in the world and this skill was duly recognised by gifts of camels and watches from Arabian princes, while the rest of the doctors were given boxes of Quality Street.

Henry went into treatment. This involved daily visits to the radiotherapy department located in the basement of the hospital, a vista of sweeping corridors decorated with the occasional cranky IKEA print, dazzlingly lit fish tanks and a single forlorn plastic rubber plant.

"It's just like having an X-ray!" he boomed.

"You don't feel anything. You wait your turn for treatment, go into the treatment room, SHE takes you there, you get on the treatment couch, you're lined up with sort of lasers so the beams go to the right place. Then, SHE leaves you there. A voice comes on the tannoy telling you to hold still. And it's over."

Henry was glowing in his enthusiasm to describe the ease of the process. He was four weeks into treatment and he had no trouble at all. But the doctor noticed that he wasn't dying his hair anymore, his roots were showing, white. The treatment was affecting him. His focus had changed.

"Towards the end of treatment you might notice some side effects from the radiotherapy. You can develop frequency and when you pee, it may sting. It's just like cystitis."

"Never had it." said Henry.

"I am not a girl just in case you hadn't noticed."

The doctor ignored the comment, hoping that this indicated that Henry was getting back on form. He explained about the short term side effects of radiotherapy, having already discussed the long term problems of impotence and damage to the rectum which can cause bleeding.

"You can also get diarrhoea. This lasts about a fortnight and gradually wears off. With modern radiotherapy techniques though, you might have no side effects at all."

"I should be so lucky!"

And Henry stomped off to find his chauffeur.

Henry did just fine. There were no problems at all. It had been a breeze and he told the doctor at his outpatient appointment.

"Don't know what the fuss was all about."

Over the next five years Henry came regularly to clinic. He had his PSA measured every time and levels remained extremely low. The PSA levels tell us what is happening to Henry's cancer. Although PSA is a very poor test for the detection of prostate cancer, it's a great test for following the course of the disease once the diagnosis has been established.

Henry changed in some ways. He never did use hair dye again. That said something about his view of himself. But he remained ebullient and challenging. He was fun.

The longer that PSA levels remain very low, the better the outcome is likely to be. But unfortunately there is no such thing as being all right forever for every single patient. For some patients relapse can come late ... but the later it comes, the better the outlook should be. Then, if PSA levels do increase, the rate of increase, the doubling time of the PSA result, tells us what the outlook should be. Doubling times of less than three months are associated with a poor outlook and longer doubling times, with a good outlook.

Statistics for survival come from analyses of the clinical course of many hundreds of patients, but these statistics give life chances for the average person, and the average person does not exist of course. Cancer survival chances when requested by the patient from the doctor give that patient an idea of life expectancy but that idea, although a truth, is not necessarily the truth for the individual patient.

"Please tell me doctor, I want to know."

"Six months."

And the days are scratched off on the wall calendar and the patient gets to six months and then nine months and isn't dead.

"Why haven't I died then?"

"I did tell you ..."

"I have wasted my time ... I would have been a lot more cheerful if I hadn't known."

"We just can't tell. We don't have a direct line to the Almighty. "

So back to Henry. Five years have gone by and his PSA test result had suddenly moved up to 7.2ng/ml.

"That's not good is it?"

Henry smiled and there was something satisfied in the smile. It was as if it had seemed to Henry that the result had confirmed his view all along as to the outcome. Although he saw death in the results of his blood test, it appeared that it almost felt good to him, that he'd been right in his judgement.

"So what you going to do about it?"

"I ..."

"I know what you're going to tell me. I'm not bloody stupid. You're going to say hormones aren't you? I am not having any of them blasted things. That's it I am not having them. They make you grow tits and your penis ends up shrivelled like a bloody corkscrew. I'm not going through with that. It's not bloody worth it."

That really isn't what hormonal therapy does. It can cause impotence but the penis doesn't shrivel and you don't grow breasts. Twenty or thirty years ago men with prostate cancer were treated with hormonal therapy using female hormones and castration. This did cause those side effects. But treatment has changed and there are modern alternatives available. Female hormone treatment with a drug called diethylstilboestrol is banned in some European countries because it also causes blood clots and heart attacks, but unfortunately is still available in the UK.

Henry crossed his legs and arms and swivelled around in the chair to face the door. He turned to glare at Stella and scowled at her with palpable hatred. And in that glance he was saying

'Why me, why not her?'

"It's not what we do. In this situation, there is no rush to treat ..."

"Yes there bloody well is a rush to treat. I am not dying from this bloody thing."

" ... It's not dangerous and early treatment doesn't provide any survival benefit ..."

"Rubbish."

"Honestly Henry ... The levels are not dangerous and the current teaching is that hormone treatment can be delayed, with the advantage of conserving life quality until PSA levels reach around 20 or 30. If the patient is anxious as a result of rising PSA levels, well, that also is an indication for treatment."

"You are bloody well right I am anxious. I want something and I want it now. But I am not having your hormones"

"How about if we do some scans, see how things are and check the PSA again."

"OK. I'll have that."

One week later, Henry was back in the consulting rooms. He had had the scans done, a CT scan, a bone scan and an MRI. All the test results were normal. Nothing abnormal could be seen.

But the repeat PSA test had given a reading of 32.

"So where is it then?"

The doctor explained that the cancer was present in microscopic form and just couldn't be seen given the limits of technology which images body organs but gives no clues as to what's going on at the level of single cells. Henry wanted to face his enemy, he wanted to know where the cancer was, because knowing it allowed him to understand it. Not knowing where it was ...

"So how come it wasn't cured? How come it takes so long for it to show itself again?"

"In many ways it's a good thing that it takes so long to show itself. It means that the tumour has grown very slowly. It's likely that the tumour was outside of the prostate in microscopic form right at the start of your illness."

"I see. So you are telling me that all that I went through wasn't worthwhile."

"No ... you might have had to deal with an even worse situation if we hadn't organised treatment."

The doctor realised as he used the word 'we' that he was being defensive. Doctors always resort to the plural form when they are against a wall.

"Henry. The PSA has gone up to 32."

Stella leaned in to the desk,

"Chemotherapy? Couldn't he have chemotherapy instead?"

After a little start of surprise at the idea, the doctor thought about it and considered that he would be willing to try it. It was extremely, completely, over and beyond unconventional but if that's what they wanted ...

"The usual is hormonal treatment."

"Not having it and that's that."

After a bit of a struggle to accept the unconventional the doctor said …

"As long as you know that this isn't the usual thing to do, I am willing to give it a go."

Henry had six courses of treatment. He had a cold cap on during the chemotherapy infusions, which prevented him losing his hair. The cold cap looks a bit like an old fashioned hair dryer. It works by reducing blood flow to the scalp and this reduces the flow of chemotherapy in the blood stream to the hair follicles. That's how hair loss is prevented.

Some doctors forget about the effects of chemotherapy on hair in men, not thinking it important, but it is, and Henry wanted to keep his rim of hair. He liked it. It was important to him. And losing it identified him as a cancer patient. He didn't want that at all. He didn't want to be pitied on the golf course, consoled at his club, gloated at by his commercial rivals. He wanted to be the same, the same as everyone else at the dinner party.

Henry was counselled about the effects of chemotherapy but he looked at his nails during the discussion and then out of the window at a vista of the car park. He seemed very interested in the car park.

So Henry had chemotherapy just as Stella suggested and this was an approach that few doctors would condone. But amazingly it worked. Henry's PSA came smack down to normal and Stella was notionally promoted to research associate at the hospital.

Henry came to clinic every two months. He had blood tests a week before each visit. He phoned for the results before he came to clinic so that he could be prepared. Henry hated surprises. And more than anything hated surprises about his health. After a period of three months from the completion of chemotherapy Henry's PSA had started to go up. He had received the news about the reading without comment on the phone but there were comments in the clinic.

"So what are you bloody well going to do? Do you mean to say that I have had all that bloody chemo for bloody nothing? It's bloody rubbish. RUBBISH."

Henry's decibels had reached Concord level. He was on the edge of his chair, fist punching the air, angry, pissed off more than anyone outside a bull ring facing a matador could ever be pissed off.

It seemed to the doctor that he had had this conversation before.

"HOW CAN IT GO FROM NOTHING TO 30 IN THREE WEEKS?"

The doctor knew how it could do that. It could do that if the tumour was in free fall growth. And the situation would become out of control if no hormonal treatment brake was being applied. It meant that the situation had changed, things were grave, and the doubling time of the PSA test result spelt really bad news for Henry.

There was Henry, angry, railing against fate, hating everything and everyone. It was good in a way that his feelings were so externalised, meant that he was dealing with the situation and would settle down, and come to terms with his things. The patients who seemed calm, accepting, placid, these were the patients to worry about. These were the people that had real trouble. Henry would be fine in the end. And it was 'end' that we were facing if the rate of change of PSA continued.

"I think that you need treatment."

"You are dammed right I do. But is there any alternative to hormonal therapy?"

There wasn't in the doctor's opinion.

"What about other opinions? You aren't the only doctor on the planet."

For many doctors, requests for second opinions are undermining, indicative of failure, unacceptable. For some, it's not a problem. They are secure in their abilities, comfortable in themselves, accepting of the challenge of loss of confidence. For many doctors, it's a relief that a patient wants another opinion because that opinion will usually confirm their own management view and also spreads the load of responsibility for their patient's fate.

"What about America? There must be some great doctors there."

Did it matter to the doctor that he was implying that his own doctor was of no importance?

"Yes Henry. Would you like me to refer you to a good doctor?"

Henry relaxed.

"Yes."

"New York?"

"Yes. Stella can come and keep me company. Might let her go shopping …

"Mind you, she'll have to spend her own money. I am not paying for anything."

One of the world's most significant cancer hospitals is the Memorial Hospital in New York. Standards are high. That's where Henry went.

"How was it Henry?"

"Wasn't that great.

"Not much different from here. They took your credit card from you when you went through the door, made you repeat every test that you ever had and then said the same as you said. I got my black Amex card back with a bite out of it.

"OK doc. Let's bring it on …

"So let's get on with it. I don't want to die you know.

" …Not that I am scared of dying.

"…It's just that … Stella won't know what to do with herself … when I am gone …"

Chapter 8
Why Me?

It's rational for the man or woman who has been given a cancer diagnosis to wonder why they have got the wretched thing. It's a natural response. And we respond rationally to our diagnosis by looking for the causes of our cancer in the life that we lead. We wonder if it is the air that we breathe. Is it our genes or is it our environment? Have we got cancer because of something bad that we have done, that we really shouldn't have done? Whatever it is, whatever the cause, cancer seems like retribution. Could it be stress or is it depression? Is it a virus or bacteria? Is it a lack of exercise or repressed anger? Whatever has done it, I have got it. Why is it me? What have I done to get this ghastly thing? Is it free radicals or not enough antioxidants? Is it the food that we eat or is it food additives? Is it microwaves or electricity pylons, is it mobile phones or radiation? They are all grand suspects in the conspiracy theory that surrounds the causes of cancer. In turn all of the suspects are brought up before a brooding jury and inspected in great detail for the villains that they are.

The consultant sits in the hospital consulting room, glamorously pitted white walls and a Formica topped desk, examination couch topped with a blue paper roll and a neatly folded blanket. What a beautiful place hospital consulting rooms are. There is a medical student by his side and they sit with Jack and Jo.

Jack has been sent up by his GP for a second opinion. He went to his GP a couple of months back with a story of

J. Waxman, *The Elephant in the Room*,
DOI 10.1007/978-0-85729-895-9_8,
© Springer-Verlag London Limited 2012

indigestion. He is 42 and hadn't been to the doctor before. He's tall with short grey hair, blue suit, button down open necked shirt. His legs are crossed and he leans forward in his chair to tell his story. Jo, his wife, is a 'footballer's wife', pretty, streaked blonde hair, short skirt and bling. Jo had made him go along to his GP because she was fed up with him whinge-ing about his belly ache and tired of him not doing anything to sort himself out.

So she told him and under orders, off he went to the GP. Now GPs don't usually see men in their surgerys until they are 72 years old and mortally sick. Men are like that; they don't go to doctors. It's something to do with the male idea of what a man is. Women are different of course. They are medi-calised, they have to be. They have to be for themselves and their children. They are medicalised by the necessity of their periods, and fertility. So when a man goes to a doctor, that doctor generally takes the visit seriously and scrutinises the patient and his symptoms with care and a morbid eye.

Jack sits in the GP's surgery, flicks through the copies of *House and Garden*, looks at the models in the worn copy of *Vogue* and wonders if they'd go out with him for a beer, or a Tequila Sunrise … if they'd prefer a cocktail to a beer. He hadn't realised it was possible to spend £855 on a pair of red stilettos. Jack crosses his legs and peers at the receptionist, who has ignored him preferring the wonders of the Argos catalogue to any interaction with patients. The red digital display beeps and

'NEXT PATIENT CONSULTING ROOM 5', tramples across the screen.

There is nobody else in the waiting room so Jack, who is clearly the next patient, brushes yesterday's almond croissant crumbs from his trousers, gets up and walks along a carpeted corridor to the doctor's office.

Of course the GP has half moon spectacles; it's in the job description. The doctor peers over those spectacles looking his patient up, then down, up and then side to side. It's not the some thing that one would do socially because such a depth of intensity might be considered a curious perversion, but here in the consulting room, it is a way of life! Doctors are trained that way, trained to look for signs in the way that we walk and talk, breathe and speak. Most good doctors work intuitively taking their diagnoses from a moment's review of the patient. Just a moment and the whole of the patient's life is there, sketched out, complete. The GP peers into Jack's life and knows that something is up.

So Jack's belly ache and Jack the person become taken up in a process that moves from blood tests and an X ray to a request for an endoscopy, where a flexible telescopic tube is inserted through the mouth, to examine the contents of the upper bowel. From the moment of the visit to the GP, Jack had become a patient. He was no longer Jack in Human Resources, Jack the father, Jack the son, husband and friend. He is Jack the patient. The patient with problems, symptoms, troubles, an illness to have and to hold, treatment to be given, a man with a chance of survival.

Jack arrived at the hospital for the endoscopy. He reported to the ward and was shown his bed by the ward clerk. He was asked to change into pyjamas. Jack lay down on the hard bed in his best pyjamas. They were new pyjamas. They were his only set of pyjamas. He hadn't had a pair of pyjamas in his adult life. They had a nice wide blue stripe to them. Jo had bought them for him when she heard that he was to have hospital tests.

'You'll need these darling,' she'd said.

She was right. She never normally called him darling. That worried Jack more than all the doctors and all the tests had ever worried him. Darling.

They'd put some numbing spray in the back of his throat. Then they shoved a big black tube the size of a hosepipe into his mouth and he'd gagged. So they'd decided that he would have to be put to sleep for the endoscopy, put a needle in a vein in the back of his hand and given him a short acting anaesthetic. He'd been told to count to 10, but had only counted to 6 when nothingness struck and he was anaesthetised.

The doctors peered down the endoscope and had seen a white fist shaped lump poking out from the smooth pink surface of the stomach. The lump shouldn't have been there. It was clearly a tumour. The endoscopist twiddled with his endoscope controls. A biopsy forceps emerged from the end of the scope and he snipped at the tumour's surface. A caterpillar bite sized snip. A little spout of blood flared from the biopsy site and then stopped. The biopsies had been taken to confirm the suspicions of the endoscopist. The biopsies were put in a transparent plastic jar filed with formalin. Formalin is a fluid that smells curiously of rotten fish, alcoholic fish. The little specimens swam in a formalin sea.

In the hospital's pathology laboratory, the material from Jack's stomach was preserved in formalin, then embedded in wax, layered in the thinnest, finest slices on to a glass microscope slide, chemically fixed to that slide and finally stained with a legion of obscure dyes that help the pathologist distinguish cancer from normal tissue. Examined under the microscope cancer cells look wilder and more disordered than normal cells. If you were looking for a comparison then compare hair that's just been cut, washed, and styled at Kieran's Styleezey Hair Salon in Crawford Street, with a toupee that's been left without conditioner, wild and free, on a salty Ibiza beach for two months.

The biopsies had shown a tumour at the upper end of Jack's stomach.

Gastric cancer and only half way through life. Didn't seem to be fair. Wasn't fair at all. Jack thought that it must have been something that he had brought on himself.

So back to the consulting room with its lovely walls.

Jack leaned forward in his chair, touched his hand to his cheek and said,

"Is it something that I have done? Why is it me?"

As the consultant looks at Jack, he sees a life unravelled before him, imagines his home and his work, his friends and his kids. The consultant sees the vista of his patient's days, the garage where he keeps his car, his outings to the Footie, his schools and his work. The consultant from small and subtle clues sees what faces his patient and think of his end. And whether he is right, whether he is wrong, he thinks that he knows him.

And for the good consultant, his answers to the patients' questions should be tailored to the man. The good consultant must guess at what his patient wishes to know and can cope with knowing, understand from the subtext of his patient's conversation what he wants from his consultant. And the consultant must make his patient comfortable with his ways as a doctor and to do so he must mirror his patient's language and his manner. The consultant must find metaphors that his patient will understand, pace his words, and put his imagery into the frames that are his patient's property. The consultant becomes a mirror for his patient and in that mirror his patient will take comfort. We take comfort in what we know. The familiar is what we want, not the wild and not the alien.

But the consultant cannot say what he is really thinking.

In many ways the consultation with a cancer specialist is like a conversation with a therapist. Great care is needed in the doctor's manner and style, for every inference is drawn from the nuance of a look or pause. The conversation must in every detail be sensitive, drawing from life experiences, radar on.

So in the traditional manner of the therapist, the consultant sensing Jack's fears says,

"Do you think that it is something that you might have done that's caused the cancer?"

And Jack, who clearly has also had therapy, smiles.

So the consultant continues.

"When anything significant happens in our lives we look for causes for our conditions. We look at our lifestyle, we examine our diet. We think about trauma, emotional, physical, we consider our psychiatric histories, depression, guilt. We consider the food that we have eaten, the bugs that we might have caught, wonder about our genes, wonder about every aspect of our days."

It is not clear that the ponderousness of the consultant's words precisely mirrored Jack's style.

How about physical trauma? Had Jack's cancer come from any injury, he asks?

The easiest way to explain this possible link is by looking at the example of women with breast cancer. The woman who has breast cancer remembers that she hurt her breast a few months ago. Walking into a restaurant, she caught her breast on a door handle. She tells the doctor about this episode. She thinks that the bruising sparked off her cancer. It is common for patients to think in this way. But there is no evidence that cancer can be caused by a single injury. Rather, in the flailing around that we do to explain what has happened, we cast back to any significant event in our lives to explain the process. For some conditions there is evidence that repeated injury can lead to the beginnings of a cancer. The damage of the sun's rays causes melanomas and other skin cancers. Rarely, chronic ulceration or repeated injury to the same site can be linked to a cancer. But there are very few examples of physical trauma that can cause cancers. There is no link between trauma and any common cancer.

What about psychiatric histories? Jack wonders if there is a link with mood.

There may be … There is a husband and he has been unfaithful to his wife. The affair finishes, but the effect on his wife was the deepest hurt. She became very badly depressed. She stayed at home, she kept to her bed, wouldn't wash, wouldn't eat, couldn't manage the kids. He got her to the doctors and the doctor prescribed antidepressants and arranged for counselling sessions. The depression lifted after many bad months, the marriage continued, staggering on, reeling from hard rock to hard rock. The memory of infidelity was always there, rearing up, accusations and tears sparked by the littlest perturbation. In her 60s, she developed colon cancer and she told him when she was dying that it was his fault. The hurt that he had caused had burned and caused the growth. The memory of his infidelity, the scar of guilt that he bore, lived for ever in him.

There is some truth in her accusation that he had caused her cancer. There have been many examinations of the importance of a psychiatric history in the subsequent development of cancers. It was shown in the 1980s that there is an association between a previous history of depression and the development of breast cancer. The link is slight. No other type of cancer has been shown to be associated with any other psychiatric illness.

Was it something that Jack had eaten? Had his cancer been caused by diet?

There is a very strong correlate between diet and cancer. Overall if one assesses the major cancers ... breast, the commonest cancer of women and prostate, the commonest cancer of men, then the risk of getting these cancers is reduced by 50% in vegetarians. Simple stuff! Fish based diets are protective and so are diets rich in yellow beans such as soya. Diets that have a high content of smoked foods or dairy produce are conducive to cancer development. Not so good for those of us who love smoked salmon and bacon. Is there a life without a smoked salmon bagel? And as Lenny Bruce said,

'Bacon ... it's the only kosher part of the pig.'

These findings about the importance of diet come from a huge body of epidemiological work. The best of these studies have arcane titles such as 'The China Study', the 'Netherlands Dietary Analysis'. Do these works take your fancy? How about 'Cancer on Five Continents'? All hardly racy, all rather obtuse, but all amazingly important works. And in these studies scientists have looked at the diets of thousands of normal people over many years and linked their diets to cancer.

There is more evidence, evidence taken from studies of mass migration. In the 1880s there were large scale migrations of Japanese to the United States. In Japan, there is a surprisingly low level of breast and prostate cancer. Over the next two generations of migrants, called the Isie and the Nisei, the incidence of these cancers rose, gradually reaching equivalence to their Caucasian neighbours. Cancers of the breast and prostate became half as common in the Isie as in Caucasians and reached equivalence in the Nisei. The Japanese generations had not intermarried, their gene base had not changed, but what had altered was their diet, from fish based to meat based, and this is the link.

Knowing all this, are cancer doctors vegetarians? No. We have coruscatingly high rates of alcoholism and smoking, with the poorest diets and the worst of life styles.

Jack has stomach cancer. What has caused this?

It would seem obvious that gastric cancer might have a dietary cause. This is the case. Stomach cancer is strongly linked to diet or to be more specific to preservatives and to food preservation.

Now here's a magic moment where a long haired conspiracy theorist can start to get excited. Great ... it's the industrial military complex at last, poisoning us for a fast buck. We were right all along!

Hold on folks. Sorry to dent your delight. Actually the incidence of stomach cancer has fallen over the years and this is largely because of food additives and better food preservation. Food, when it decays, produces free radicals. Free radicals are charged particles that by chemical reaction cause damage to normal tissue and this damage is one of the steps in the molecular history of the development of cancer. Better food preservation, fresher food, has reduced free radical production and limited the chemical reactions that follow. The use of additives, the addition of artificial preservatives has further brought down the availability of free radicals, and acted as scavengers for those bad boy free radicals.

So what has Jack left as a likely cause for his cancer? He is a young man with cancer and in the young the likely causes are not environmental, more likely they are genetic. But the genetic cause of Jack's cancer is something about which we are awesomely ignorant. We just dunnoh! There is so much of which we are ignorant, so much that we will never know and this is a frustration for our patient as we cannot explain and we have to leave him with a riddle as to the reasons for his condition.

The philosopher Susan Sontag wrote about cancer and its causes in a great book called 'Illness as Metaphor'.

Susan Sontag compares current views as to cancer and its causes to views held by the Victorians about TB. In the 19th century, TB was a mystery. No one understood how it came and no one understood why it came. In the 19th century patients with TB would ascribe their condition to an excess of humours, to diet, to mood. They took bizarre cures, dieted, blamed themselves for their condition, they struggled and died. Then a wonderful man … Koch, came with a microscope. Koch spotted the TB bacillus through his long lens and the mysteries of TB were solved.

So will it be with cancer. But cancer is not one disease but many illnesses. We can explain the causes of some cancers, we know the genes, and we know the mutations in the genes but for a complex of diseases which bear a generic title, 'Cancer', the explanations and revelations will come a bit at a time.

But at this point in the early 21st century we are ignorant of the causes of 90% of the cancers that affect us and this the consultant explains to Jack …

"So Jack … what do you think?"

Jack's eyes redden rational for the and well. Jo reaches for him and he pushes her away.

"If you don't know what's caused this, how the hell am I meant to go on?"

And the consultant shifts in his seat and says,

"I haven't an answer …"

Jack blew his nose and wiped his eyes. He shrugged, looked up and said,

"But I know that I have to go on."

Jo's arm comes back and this time it's not brushed away.

Chapter 9
How Do They Know What I've Got?

The diagnosis of cancer is virtually always made from a patient's initial history and confirmed by scans and a biopsy. The scans and the biopsy are generally a finessing of what is already clear from the history. A patient will give a description of pain or bleeding, weight loss or cough. From these descriptions, the cause for the symptoms is generally obvious to the grey haired pompous old fart of a clinician who thinks he knows everything but, if he is any good at all, is frequently astonished by how little he knows, and is neither pompous nor an old fart.

Experience and sensitivity to the nuances of each patient's presentation are critical facilities that define the good doctor. The clever clinicians' radar is always on. Practice makes almost perfect, but the best of doctors are aware that their practice is imperfect, and needs refinement. Although the clinician's diagnosis is made from a patient's symptoms the diagnosis comes to proof through tests and biopsies, objective evidence that defines treatment and provides a prognosis.

The histories that patients recite are in many ways stereotypic. They form a pattern and these patterns are what the clinician recognises. As a medical student I was astonished … I was habitually astonished … but in this case … truly astonished by one of our teachers, Dr William Goody, who was a consultant neurologist. Dr Goody was very eminent and we all knew it. He told us of his eminence by the way he walked and the way in which he talked. The walk was a glide and the

J. Waxman, *The Elephant in the Room*,
DOI 10.1007/978-0-85729-895-9_9,
© Springer-Verlag London Limited 2012

talk a peering, peeking sort of talk that seemed to float up from his lips, roll over the edge of his spectacles and tumble down to us, mortal students, from somewhere just under the dip of his grey, grey hair.

Dr Goody taught at my medical school, University College London but also had an appointment at the National Hospital for Nervous Diseases, a hallowed place of learning. University College had been founded by Jeremy Bentham, that great reformist, Quaker, and utilitarian, founded for dissenters and non-conformists. The utilitarian belief that nothing should be of waste and everything should be of use was embodied in Bentham's bequest of his corpse to UCL, where, when I was at medical school, he sat stuffed in 18th century breeches, lace ruffle and velvet coat, seated in a sedan chair with glass doors, tucked into a corner of the entrance hall. His skull was separated from his body and looks down at the students and porters from a high point in the sedan chair.

Our teaching took the form of a classical apprenticeship where we learnt by the example of our seniors, when we bothered to take time out from our bouts of high jinks and they bothered to take time out from Harley Street.

We were placed around Dr Goody in a circle of low uncomfortable chairs; he had an armchair. The armchair seemed to be on a raised dais. Ringed by medical students in short white coats, Dr Goody swept his right hand through his hair and then spent some moments inspecting his manicure.

"Who is going to present the case to me?"

Ashley Grossman sat forward and looked keen. Ashley was keen. Ashley was very keen. He had married my cousin Susan. Ashley was clever. Ashley was very clever. He went on to win the university gold medal given to the top medical student at graduation and eventually became Professor of Endocrinology at Bart's Hospital.

"I'd like to present Mrs Millie Friedman's case to you, Dr Goody."

"Thank you Grossman … that'll be quite enough."

And Dr Goody then went on to give the story himself, telling us of Mrs Friedman's age and life, her medical details and her medications, her symptoms and their investigations, her family history and her past medical history. And then on to the dénouement of Mrs F's current problem, finishing by bringing everything together in a final sweep through current research in the area of her diagnosis of dementia.

Dr Goody stopped. He rose from his chair and left the room. It had been a tour de force of intuition and perception. We were breathless in our amazement. How had he managed to deduce Mrs F's condition from just a name? He was brilliant. How had he done it? Many of the more cynical of us thought that he had known all along about Mrs F, having seen her a week back in the out patients clinic, but some of us felt that it was likely that he had not cheated but had given us the benefit of his sentience and skill, abilities that took origin in his own unique ability and from his years of clinical experience. We felt that he had made the diagnosis from her name. Her first name had given Dr Goody a clue as to her age and from this clue he had worked out the illnesses that would be likely in a woman of Mrs Friedman's years. And from her surname … we thought that this clue had pointed Dr Goody towards the neurological diseases specific to Central European Jews. So he had put the clues together and made the diagnosis just from her name.

The 68 year old smoker goes to his GP with a cough and phlegm. The phlegm has streaks of blood in it and the doctor doesn't have to be a genius to know that the man has lung cancer. Any other cause is highly unlikely. It's like GCSE medicine. It's obvious but not always. There are surprises and that's why it's unbelievably important to have proof of the diagnosis.

The elderly woman has had a change in her bowel habit and from a life time of 'being regular', 'like clockwork doctor', 'I'm constipated'. She's got a bowel cancer and anything else would seem to be exceptionally unlikely.

The retired boilermaker from London's East End has chest pain and abdominal swelling and the doctor diagnoses mesothelioma.

'I've got trouble with my waterworks doc.'

'Ah. Trouble with the waterworks then you'll need a plumber.'

But seriously there could be a differential diagnosis here because not all trouble in the men's department is caused by cancer.

And the lump in my breast … You are only 33 years old so let's look on the bright side for once. Breast cancer is unusual in the young. It does happen and the lump has to be checked.

So how do doctors diagnose a cancer?

This is how a diagnosis is made, this is what happens. Here is John's story.

John came to London from the West Indies. He had left Jamaica in 1965 and came to stay with his brother in a rented flat in Notting Hill. His brother had met him as he came off the boat at Southampton, hugged him, chucked John's embarrassing cloth cap in a bin and took him home to London. John had come from the sunshine of the Islands to the city's rain and found streets paved with base metal on the borders between W8 and W9. The house was divided into 18 bed-sits. The paintwork was peeling and the window frames rotting. The house was owned by a man called Peter Rachman. Each week his brother gave the rent in cash to an unpleasant chap called Mick. Mick had no neck and a camel coloured cashmere coat. Mick made sure that the rent came in on the button, the real horn button.

John had been trained as a motor mechanic and after a couple of months got a job in a garage under the railway arches in Ladbroke Grove. After a couple of years he had found a nice wife and moved to Harlesden where the children came and went.

John smoked, had done since he was 13 years old. Over the previous two or three months he had right sided chest pain that came and went. It was a strange sort of pain that was worse with a big breath or a cough. And he had a cough, mostly dry but sometimes he brought up a little plug of mucus, green or white. He coughed one morning at breakfast and the sputum was blood streaked. His wife Serena looked at him anxiously.

"Don't like your cough John. You've had it for months now. It's not getting better. It's really not"

So the two of them went to his GP, and she told the details of his story to the doctor. It's usually like that; the men unable to give the specifics of their problem, unable to recount the time and the order of things, relying on their partners for the detail. The GP listened and then asked if John smoked.

"Not really doc. ... stopped now."

This stopping smoking is an alarm call to the doctor. It happens to older people when they think that something serious is affecting them. The fags go straight into the bin when the smoker thinks that he's got cancer. So when he finds out that his patient has stopped smoking, the doctor knows it's important.

"John I think you need an X ray."

"Is serious doc?"

"Not certain ... but we'd best check."

The doc is certain. He knows that there will be a nasty little spot somewhere on the X-ray, a sure sign that there is a tumour causing that irksome cough and tiresome chest pain. The chest pain comes from one of two causes. The lungs have no nerves that detect pain, but the lining of the lung, which is called the pleura does have pain sensors. So it could be that the tumour is touching the pleura and causing the pain. The alternative possibility is that the cancer has spread to John's ribs and that is the reason for his pain. The ribs themselves also have no pain fibres and pain that takes its origins from the ribs comes from sensory nerve fibres in the covering of the ribs, which is called the periosteum. Characteristically, pain that increases with a cough or a deep breath generally comes from the ribs. Secondary tumours have spun away from the primary tumour in the lung, travelling in the blood stream and seeding in the ribs. There, when they have reached a large enough size to push the periosteum away from the ribs that it covers, the secondary cancer will cause nerve fibres to fire and pain to be felt.

The doctor is not surprised when the results of John's X-ray are faxed to him from the X-ray department of the local hospital. It is standard procedure and good practice for the results of grossly abnormal X-rays to be sent directly to the GP.

John is called back to the surgery. He's there now with Serena. The two of them, sitting with the doctor, anxious, wondering why he's called them to the surgery, but of course, knowing in their hearts the reason for their recall.

"There's nothing to worry about ..." said their GP.

Translation: *'There's everything to worry about.'*

"It's a little spot on the lung."

Translation: *'There's a huge spot on the lung.'*

"It could be anything really, an infection, an old scar."

Translation: *'Time's up. It's cancer.'*

In the UK if a GP suspects a cancer diagnosis then he refers the patient to see a hospital specialist under the suspected cancer two week wait guideline. The form is faxed and the appointment made.

For John, the first hospital appointment is with a chest physician. John's story is told again. By this time the details of the story have been firmed up and like most men, given a decent period of time and a following wind, John has just about got the gist of what had been happening to him. Serena doesn't have to interrupt all that often, only once or twice to remind him of dates.

The chest physician then examines John. John stripped to his pants and lay down on one of those lovely rolls of paper that stick to one's back in the summer and are merely uncomfortable in the winter. Dr Goldberg is kind of sweaty in all weathers, rather round, acne scarred, bow tie. He starts with John's general appearance.

'Good enough.' he thinks.

' ... This one might be a runner. He might just make it.'

Then he takes John's hand. This feels a bit alarming to John. He's hasn't held hands with a man since childhood.

Dr Goldberg turns John's hand in his hand. He looks at John's nails first.

'Hmmm. Curved. But does he have clubbing?'

There is a particular curve to the nail bed that is caused by some cancers. The curvature is called clubbing and results from the secretion by the cancer into the blood stream of a chemical with the peculiar property of changing the shape of the nails. This chemical is made by a particular type of lung cancer, the variant that is operable.

John's finger nails are clubbed. So Dr Goldberg has made his diagnosis and more than that, in the first moments of his examination is formulating a plan for John's treatment.

Dr Goldberg looks at the colour of John's nails and then examines John's palms. He sees that they are of normal colour which tells him that it is likely that John is not anaemic. Patients with cancer become anaemic. The anaemia has many causes in cancer patients but the commonest reason is a non specific reduction in the rate at which the bone marrow forms red blood cells. This is the result of the cancer making yet another chemical that it dumps into the blood stream which then circulates to the bone marrow and switches off blood cell production.

'Hmm … not anaemic. He might 'do' then. He just might make it.'

Dr Goldberg thinks that at this point John's tumour might not be too advanced as to preclude him from surgery. In other words, he might be in that small group of patients whose tumours are contained enough to be removed.

Then that nice Dr G scratches his cheek. Fortunately it's not his bottom cheek and goes on to feel in John's armpits and around John's neck. It's there in the armpits and neck that lymph nodes appear. These are glands that sometimes become enlarged when you've a cold, but that also become enlarged because of spread of cancer cells to these nodes.

Dr G says to John.

"Fine so far. There are no nodes."

And John doesn't know what the hell the doctor is talking about. What are nodes for goodness sakes? But he smiles enthusiastically because the doctor seems to be giving him good news and good news is all that we want.

Dr G asks John to sit up and watches him breathe,

"In and out for me."

He looks for symmetry of chest movement, the position of the trachea, and at John's general state of health. Then he taps at the chest in an ordered way listening to the echoes of his fingers, the depth of the drumbeat telling him of the state of the tissue beneath. Dull for fluid and solid structures, tympanic for normal lung. He leans over John and listens to his breathing and John's feels the breath of the doctor on his chest, smells the garlic and the aftershave. There shouldn't be garlic on a doctor's breath and there certainly shouldn't be fluid in a patient's chest. If there is fluid then that's a bad, bad sign.

"Almost done. Just going to feel your liver and bang your bones."

John doesn't like the idea of Dr Goldberg feeling his liver. He's alright with the bone banging though!

'Hmmm … bit big that! So he might not make it after all.'

Dr G worries that John may have spread of his cancer to his liver. But there are other causes of liver enlargement and they come in glass bottles.

"Excuse me Sir, are you a drinking man?"

This 'Sir' thing is an antiquated formulaic way that older middle class doctor have with working class men. They speak down pretending to speak up and it's yucky.

"Not really doc."

"John, tell the doctor the truth," says Serena.

And John's Friday nights at the Harlesden Social and Saturday nights at the Sunshine Club are explained to Dr Goldberg.

John gets dressed and Dr Goldberg talks about the tests that he needs.

"Anything you say doc."

Surprisingly, in these modern times of choice and options, most patients would rather be told what to do, than be confronted with options. Options may be indicative of therapeutic uncertainty to the patient and what is needed at this time of great stress is certainty. Because with certainty there is comfort and hope, and with hope …

A few years ago on a ward round, with its trail of nurses and junior doctors, I discussed the options for treatment with a woman photographer who had metastatic breast cancer. She listened from her bed as I explained that one chemotherapy option would give her this or that percentage chance of cure, but would have side effects which I described. I then went on to talk of the other options for treatment and their side effects. She listened solemnly and said

"Let me think about it."

The ward round moved on, and as we walked away, she called Mark Bower, the most junior of the doctors, back to her bedside,

"Listen Mark!" she said,

"What should I do? If he doesn't know, how am I supposed to know?"

I take my car to Humphrey the mechanic to be serviced. I have been going to Humph for many years. He always gets the car sorted out. We have no tense discussions about the variants of brake pads, no agonies over the species of engine oil. He just does the job. I leave the car with Humph in the morning and pick it up completely cured in the evening. It feels good knowing that he knows what to do and is so entirely reliable.

But cars are not patients. From the doctor's view, the way has to be worked out for each person that he sees. For every patient is clearly an individual with different needs from the next patient. So, for each man and each woman a different interaction is required, with different levels of information issued about options and prognoses. Some patients will say that they want to know everything but they really don't and others will say that they want to go a day at a time, but really want to hear about every detail. The doctor has to be aware of subtexts and sensitivity makes for a great doctor.

So John is sent for more X rays and scans. Scans of his soft tissues, liver and lungs … a CT scan, and scans of his bones … a bone scan. A CT scan uses multiple X-rays to build up a composite computerised image of internal organs. A bone scan involves the injection of a radioisotope into the blood. The isotope homes to bone and the emissions of the isotope from bone are picked up by sensors. The intensity of the signal shows whether or not there is spread of the cancer to the bones.

The CT scan reveals that John has a small operable tumour and the bone scan is negative. 'Negative'; this is doctor speak for no spread of cancer to the bones. Remarkably, 'positive' results, which one would imagine to be a good thing, is ia bad thing and indicates that the cancer has spread.

John has a bronchoscopy. A flexible tube which is called a bronchoscope is inserted into the mouth under either local anaesthetic or a general anaesthetic. The bronchoscope is then pushed down into the throat, from the throat to the larynx, from the larynx to the trachea and then to the two main bronchi. Beyond the two main bronchi are the sub-divisions of the bronchial tree that climb down deep into the lungs.

The Bronchoscopy Suite. This is Dr Goldberg's happy corner. He likes it there. It's his kingdom, the only safe place in the hospital. Peace of a sort and a cup of tea and biscuits at the end of his bronchoscopy list, if he's not had too many tantrums. The nurses are nice to him there and yes, one or two of the nurses are actually quite attractive. But there, what would he do with them? They are half his age. He's become invisible to 20 year olds, not that he ever was much of a dish on wheels.

John's mouth yawns wide and the bronchoscope slips down and down. Then there it is just at the point where the larynx splits into two. Dr G sees the tumour. Its knobbly and cream coloured, measures about 2 cm across and it's oozing a little blood. He looks at the point of its origin with great care. It's operable if it's more than a certain distance from where the larynx splits in two and not if it's less. It's ok. It is beyond the critical point. Dr G biopsies the tumour removes the bronchoscope and goes off to his cuppa, no biscuits today which makes him feel unloved and grumpy.

The biopsy takes a few days to process. John's case is then reviewed at a Multidisciplinary Team meeting where John's case will be discussed by all other specialty doctors who are involved with lung cancer management, the surgeons and pathologists, the radiologists and the medical oncologists, the radiotherapists and the chest physicians, the juniors and the seniors. It's a good thing; and from consensus and hopefully with an evidence base, the way forward for John had been found.

Two weeks after their first hospital visit, John and Serena are in clinic with Dr Goldberg. Serena has on her Sunday church clothes and John is in his suit. Dr Goldberg thinks he's coming down with flu but he's doing his best to be a big boy and not complain too much even though he is really, really, really suffering. He's taken two paracetamol tablets, so it must be really bad. What sympathy does he get from the nurses? None. What a life.

"So how are you Sir? Recovered from the broncho-scopy?"

John's wondering why that doctor fellow isn't coming to the point.

'Why is he beating around the bush?

'Must be bad news.'

Mrs John is not breathing. She hasn't taken a breath since lunch time. She knows it's really bad. And that Dr G has confirmed it all by being pleasant to them.

Dr Goldberg continues.

"We have some news for you."

John's heart stops. It's been beating so hard and now it's had enough. Everything in him waits for the words, words that he knows, words that say …

"We have a diagnosis now. The tests have shown that you have a cancer but we think we can get it out … I am going to send you to the surgeon, if that's OK with you both? With a bit of luck … I think that you will be all right."

'There!' thought Dr Goldberg

'I think that I handled that brilliantly. Wonder if there are any Garibaldi biscuits left in the bronchoscopy suite?'

Chapter 10
Doctors and Cancer: Firewall

My mother telephoned.

"I'm worried about your father. He's not right. You know how good his memory is"

My father worked as a psychiatrist, and work was what he did. He loved his job almost as much as he loved my mother. When he retired from the National Health Service, he continued in private practice and, at the age of 76, walked to his private consulting rooms in Harley Street every darned day. He was a great "carer", taking responsibility for everyone around him, and the love that he gave in his dealings with patients made him a local celebrity. As a child, I spent a lot of my time with him in school holidays, and walking through our North London streets was the suburban equivalent of a royal procession. We'd always meet people that he'd know, and he'd stop and chat en route to the bank for his pocket money or to the tobacconists for his carton of Senior Service cigarettes and tin of four square pipe tobacco.

My father was of average height, slim and bald, with a ring of curly black hair slicked to his scalp with Brylcreme. He'd been in the Royal Army Medical Corps in the Second World War, and had been one of the doctors that had mopped up at Belsen, an experience that was with him forever. Dad had gone into general practice after military service. After we kids had grown up, he became a psychiatrist.

My father's general practice was in our house, and our house backed on to the edge of a council estate. Our garden

J. Waxman, *The Elephant in the Room*,
DOI 10.1007/978-0-85729-895-9_10,
© Springer-Verlag London Limited 2012

had trees, a lawn circled by a path, which was great for bicycle time trials. There was a trellis of tatty roses, and my chicken run, patch of purple iris and skinny potatoes. There was a willow that was great for sulking in.

At the bottom of the garden was a garage, and in the garage Dad kept his war photographs, sepia images of tanks and soldiers, and the nightmare camps with their lumpy hillocks of broken bodies.

Beyond the garden were our neighbours, the Misses Blunt, two frail spinster ladies who kept a clean and tidy house, and on the other side, and I mean the other side ... there was the Fallon family. Old Mr Fallon had spent a considerable part of his life in prison for child molestation. Out of prison, he'd spent time slouching at his garden gate, hands in the deep pocket of a baggy tweed jacket.

Our house was mock Tudor, with a curving tarmac drive and privet hedge. On the corner opposite the house was an enormous lime tree, and our front doorstep was the staging post for the victims of bloody bashes, noisy encounters between the magnetic lime and speeding cars.

So it seemed, from my mother's call, that my father had been going to work, and in his rooms he had been not been doing very much, sitting at his large oak desk amidst the books and velvet covered psychiatrist's couches. This was out of character because Dad always did "things". Mum explained that his patients had phoned, leaving telephone messages about appointments that he had not kept. Dad had become erratic about the times of his arrival and departure to work. The precision of the 8:15 start had been replaced by any old morning time, and he'd not returned home until Mum had called him.

"Well, Mum, I'll arrange for Dad to see somebody at the hospital."

I thought that he ought to see a geriatrician because geriatricians deal with older patients and specialise in the management of memory loss. My father's memory loss was quite acute and so, for that reason, I wondered whether there was a specific cause of the problem other than Alzheimer's disease. We are trained, as doctors, to look for the rare, potentially curable, causes of dementia, and these treatable dementias are usually acute in their presentations.

I phoned our hospital's geriatrics consultant, a man who had looked 60 years old at the age of 30, and continued that way until he reached retirement, when he seemed too young to retire.

"Yes, certainly, Jonathan. I'll see him."

"Well, thanks very much, Chris. When can you see him?"

"Well, I'm sure we can find an appointment in about six weeks' time."

So I spoke to my Mum about this, and she said

"I WANT HIM SEEN NOW!"

So I phoned up a rather more perceptive colleague, a neurologist, and Richard arranged to see him the next day. Scans were booked, and Dad's brain scan was horribly abnormal. He was admitted to the National Hospital for Nervous Diseases for a biopsy, under the care of the most famous neurosurgeon of the time.

Dad was at ease in hospital, and seemed relaxed with the process of being a patient; the disempowerment of a surrender to medicine that was comforting. In the ward I pulled his folder from the medical record trolley, to the grizzly gaze and prickly disapproval of three ugly nurses, and read the diagnosis, written in his notes, of a suspected glioblastoma. I flicked through the plastic sheets of brain CT scans and saw the poisonous white spider's web of the tumour's traces creeping out through the normal structures of his brain. Those images and that moment are with me now.

Dad had his biopsy the next morning, and in the afternoon, when I visited, I found him sitting in one of those horrid, unstylish, plastic covered hospital chairs; one of those chairs that is always in the same position by the patient's bedside, in every room, in every hospital in the western world. Dad had a small, square plaster slapped over his skull. My mother was with him.

"The surgeon's just been in", said my Mum.

"He told us that your father has a tumour, and then he left."

The famous surgeon had broken bad news, badly, without pausing for questions or suggesting that any treatment might be possible, or that perhaps that they might like a nice cup of tea as a consolation.

"Well, we'd better have a drink."

I'd brought a bottle of whisky to the hospital and it was in the bedside cabinet. Dad got up from his chair, and we walked together into the corridor to the water fountain because Dad liked to water his whisky. Apart from the Elastoplast on his skull, he seemed absolutely fine, quite solid in his dressing gown and comfy slippers.

"Is there anything you'd like to talk about, Dad?"

"No."

This was the sort of open ended question that I'd been taught to ask my patients, but the response that my father had given was not typical of any patient that I'd ever dealt with before. So, whisky in disposable plastic glasses in hand, we walked back into Dad's room and sat for a while, talking about the trivia that is so fundamental to the comfort of all human lives; how my children were, and how his children - my brother, sister and I - were managing at work and managing with their partners.

And then Dad said that he'd like to go home. So going home was arranged.

My parents had moved from the suburbs to a town house in a cobbled mews off Harley Street and another family had inherited the potato patch. The kitchen and dining room were downstairs, the bedrooms, sitting rooms and bathrooms were reached by narrow stairs. Dad was relatively mobile when he got home but then, over the course of the next two or three days, he found it more and more difficult to walk. My mother called me at work to say that Dad had got stuck in the bath, and there I found him, tenderly covered, warm, and amused by his situation. I helped him to his bed. Karol Sikora, beloved friend and colleague, offered to see Dad, and so off Dad went with Mum and John the Taxi Driver, to see him at the hospital.

By this time, Dad couldn't walk at all and, when out of bed, was confined to a wheelchair. His mental function was reasonably good, but his memory was poor. In the formal testing of mental function, patients are asked simple questions, such as the name of the Prime Minister, the date, or how they'd got to the hospital. They might be asked to deduct 7 serially from 100, and they might also be asked about significant events in their past lives. Dad managed the serial 7's like a Maths God, but when asked about a past event, he said,

"Your mother is my memory."

A phrase of such beauty and completeness, a phrase so redolent of love.

Dad was wheeled out of Karol's consulting room and was shunted against the wall of a hospital corridor, dehumanised, a patient like any other patient; no longer the doctor, just another sick soul.

Karol had been asked about treatment for Dad. His advice was that no radiotherapy should be given because Dad's physical state was so poor that he was unlikely to improve and might worsen with radiation treatment. This was medically the correct view, but it did seem such a terrible, terrible thing that someone should be left without any hope of improvement. There would be no way forward except the sour, stumbling path to the grave.

When I had started Oncology training, all those echoing years ago, my friend, Ian Fiertag had asked,

"What do you say to people?"

"What do you mean?"

"You know, at the end."

"Well, we have to tell them the truth."

"No, you don't. You can't do that. You must always give some hope …

"Can you imagine what it's like to be given no hope?"

And Ian's words took me completely with their truth. How can you take away all hope? With Ian's words, I imagined myself at some future time being told

"There's nothing"

And being left with, nothing.

Ian's approach is very much not the modern consensus, which is to provide everybody with the facts. I'm afraid that, in my time, I haven't always rattled the bare bones of despair. I've taken Ian's advice and always said that there was something that we could do. This approach is probably horribly wrong, but if I have made a mistake, I'm happy to take responsibility for this ghastly error.

Karol explained to my parents that the treatment for Dad's problem would involve steroids, and that radiotherapy should be reserved for when it was really necessary. He said this kindly, and Dad went home with John the Driver and Mum. When they got home, Dad was unable to walk, and John, bless him, carried him up the stairs to his bed.

The next day the Macmillan team visited, and the team included the remarkable and charismatic Rob George; Rob, the palliative care doctor. It was amazing to see the numbers of people that were involved in my father's illness, unpaid carers and nurses, doctors and all sorts. There was always somebody there, either to support my mother, or to make sure that the clinical care for my father was just right.

My beautiful brother and I abandoned work and took up residence at our parents' house. In the gloomy confines of the broom cupboard under the stairs lived a large supply of fine wine and malt whisky, presents that my father had been given by his patients. The store had grown over the years because he always drank cheap whisky and wine. I'm sure that the reason for this modesty was because he'd been brought up in a careful way, and that he was a self deprecating man, who felt that the good drink was for guests. The guests who drank the good drink were my brother and I. We stole the patient's gifts and the good whisky and fine old wine were ballast for our nerves.

Dad started treatment with steroids, and the effect was quite extraordinary. Everything improved. He was able to get out of bed and walk around the house. I followed him as he went into the sitting room. In my parents' house, the sitting room was always a special place that was kept for visitors, and not otherwise used. There were trembly antiques, nice china, silk covered Regency furniture, an ebony and brass desk and some fine, but not famous, oils.

Dad sat in the chair that his father had sat in, and we were alone together. I said ...

"Dad, I'm sorry to have given you such boochvaitik."

This is a word which, in a certain, doggerel European language, means bellyache. My father had had great pleasure in speaking in this doggerel language, which is half brother to German, to German officers at the end of the war, and I think that the German officers had not had great pleasure in having to converse with him in Yiddish.

"No. I was fine. But it wasn't so easy for your mother."

We went for a walk round the block, strolling past the terraces of wonderful Georgian and Victorian houses. It was his last walk, and he knew it. He looked around a lot, didn't speak and stumbled a little before taking my arm.

That afternoon the family came round: cousins, nephews and nieces, and his older brother, Sam. There were bridge rolls and tea. How do bridge rolls get their name? Nobody talked about Dad's illness. Everyone knew, that for him, it was the last family gathering. My daughter, Thea, blonde curls and baby podge, crawled at his knees. He picked her up and hugged her, and she was content on his lap for a long while, a long while, that is, for a baby.

My sister had been called home from South Africa and she was due to arrive in two days' time. During those two days my father's condition deteriorated. His level of consciousness changed, and he sank away from us, falling deeper and deeper into the darkness.

My father lay on his side in his bed, eyes shut, and his hand flickered across his face. It was clear that he was uncomfortable with the stubble on his cheeks. So my brother shaved him, and I was reminded of another long gone time, 30 years before, when I'd seen my father shave his father with a cut throat razor. Grandpa had been a patient in Edgware General Hospital. A few days after having kidney surgery my grandfather died from a pulmonary embolus.

Dad lay in bed, his head turned towards the window. The grey light of England rolled over the rococo mirror on my mother's dressing table, and her silver mirrored combs and brushes sparkled. His eyes were shut. There were words that came from him, words that were repeated, and repeated, and repeated. The words were …

"Roofah Shlamar."

Following the death of his parents my father had become religious, and the religion was a funny sort of religion which involved Dad saying regular daily prayers but not observing any other particular form of religious obeisance. I'm sure that he didn't believe in God. His parents had come from a shtetel, which is a word that means a Jewish village. The village was called Yarmalenitz and was in the Pale of Settlement, an area of Russia where the Jews were allowed to live after being kicked out of Germany in the 19th century. Dad's father had come to England in 1904 on a boat from the port of Kiev. I remember grandpa telling me how he'd hidden as a child in the cellars of Yarmalenitz whilst the Cossacks had stormed through the village, leaning low on their ponies, looking for Jews to spear.

And what does Roofah Shlamar mean? It comes from a prayer repeated many times daily in the Jewish Order of Prayers, where God, gets asked to 'Heal the sick.' This prayer doesn't seem to work.

Dad began to fit, little jerking movements of his face, momentary twitches of his right cheek. He was catheterised because he had lost all control of urination. Rob, the palliative care consultant, "forgot" his briefcase, leaving overnight with me that soft brown case whose contents had a street value in used notes, a street value of many thousands of pounds.

Left alone without doctors and nurses, I was the doctor and nurse for my father. When my father fitted, I opened Rob's case and drew up drugs in a syringe, chose the vein in his forearm and pushed the needle into the vein. My father's blood came into the chamber of the syringe and I emptied the syringe's contents into him.

Dad was deeply unconscious. My sister was due to return from South Africa the next morning.

Rob came again and, told of my sister's imminent arrival, gave my father an enormous dose of steroids.

Dad slept through the night and in the morning my sister rushed in from Heathrow. She ran upstairs to my parents' bedroom, and, at the rush and noise, my father awoke from his deep darkness. He opened his eyes, smiled, and said

"Hello, Chuchelel."

His pet word for my sister. Unbelievable. He'd woken up. He'd come back from death. My family cried, but their tears were silent. I didn't cry.

In my memory, he was lucid for a few more hours. He sat up in bed, propped against the pillows, listening to her news, but then, over the next few days, Dad went down into that dark cave from which there would be no exit. His breathing became intermittent and heavy, a pattern known as Cheyne-Stokes respiration that I had seen so often in my patients. This is a frightening breathing pattern for people who have had no experience of it, but in oncology, life and death is so much of a humdrum experience, that feelings become lost, and clinicians lose their emotional responses; everything leaves the doctor untouched.

As with everyone and every bright life, at a moment he was there, and at the next beat the breathing stopped. His face stiffened, all vibrant life had gone, and he was a corpse. A body, with only a distant cold relationship to the man who had been.

So Dad was dead. My uncle and I registered his death. We did so on a Sunday, visiting the Registrar of Births, Deaths and Marriages, an ironic conjunction of options, in her home in a council flat on the first floor of an estate off Lisson Grove.

Dad's grave was dug out of the cold, orange clay at Bushey Cemetery.

At Bushey Cemetery there are gravestones with the names of people who had been so splendid in the days of my child-hood. Bushey is always cold in the warmest summer, always windswept on the most tranquil of days. Bushey is desolate. A howling place. Dad's pine coffin was lowered into the earth, the line of mourners taking their turn to spade clods of clay, the sounds of the earth falling on the tinker's drum of his coffin, at first noisy, then dull.

That was it. And I never cried, but just thought 'Dad's dead'. I am sure that the reasons for this lack of emotional response to his death came from the nature of my day job, where at every moment I encounter death and tears. The only tools that I have for survival are those that wrap any sensitivity that I might have been blessed with in a deep layer of lard, so that nothing that goes on hurts.

In 2008 I met my friend, Naomi, again. Naomi, whom I hadn't seen for two decades. We'd lived together and then separated. We became close once more, and went to New York for big fun. On the plane we saw a great film, 'In Bruges' and crossing the Atlantic, looked forward to a great jaunt in Manhattan.

We caught up with our pasts, and Naomi asked

"What happened to your father?"

So I told her, in an easy listening way, the circumstances of his death but then, at the Roofe-whatever-it-was-Shlamar bit, I suddenly found myself crying. There I was, 56 years old, and blubbing. And my tears were deep and painful. It seemed that somehow defences had been breached, and my security firewall had been torched by flame. Breached, because I had been taken out of the environment where I had so carefully assembled protective walls. I should have remembered to take the walls on holiday.

When I'm next at work, I must talk to Mohamed in the University IT Computer Advice Centre about sourcing an asbestos firewall.